ROUTLEDGE LIBF
DOMESTI(

Volume 6

VIOLENCE

VIOLENCE
A Guide for the Caring Professions

R. GLYNN OWENS AND
J. BARRIE ASHCROFT

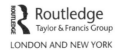

Routledge
Taylor & Francis Group

LONDON AND NEW YORK

First published in 1985 by Croom Helm Ltd

This edition first published in 2016
by Routledge
2 Park Square, Milton Park, Abingdon, Oxon OX14 4RN

and by Routledge
711 Third Avenue, New York, NY 10017

Routledge is an imprint of the Taylor & Francis Group, an informa business

British Library Cataloguing in Publication Data
A catalogue record for this book is available from the British Library

ISBN: 978-1-138-67381-6 (Set)
ISBN: 978-1-315-56168-4 (Set) (ebk)
ISBN: 978-1-138-67129-4 (Volume 6) (hbk)
ISBN: 978-1-138-67130-0 (Volume 6) (pbk)
ISBN: 978-1-315-61708-4 (Volume 6) (ebk)

Publisher's Note
The publisher has gone to great lengths to ensure the quality of this reprint but points out that some imperfections in the original copies may be apparent.

Disclaimer
The publisher has made every effort to trace copyright holders and would welcome correspondence from those they have been unable to trace.

VIOLENCE
A Guide for the Caring Professions

R. Glynn Owens
and J. Barrie Ashcroft

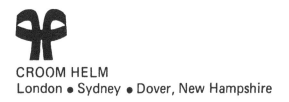

CROOM HELM
London • Sydney • Dover, New Hampshire

© 1985 R. Glynn Owens and J. Barrie Ashcroft
Croom Helm Ltd, Provident House, Burrell Row,
Beckenham, Kent BR3 1AT
Croom Helm Australia Pty Ltd, First Floor,
139 King Street, Sydney, NSW 2001, Australia

British Library Cataloguing in Publication Data

Owens, R. Glynn
    Violence: a guide for the caring professions.
    1. Violence
    I. Title II. Ashcroft, J. Barrie
    303.6'2   HM281

    ISBN 0-7099-1931-X
    ISBN 0-7099-1938-7 (Pbk)

Croom Helm, 51 Washington Street, Dover,
New Hampshire 03820, USA

Library of Congress Cataloging in Publication Data

Owens, R. Glynn.
    Violence: A guide for the caring professions.

    Bibliography: p.
    Includes index.
    1. Violence – Psychological aspects. 2. Helping
Behavior. I. Ashcroft, J. Barrie. II. Title.
RC569.5.V55094 1985   616.85'82   84-23865
ISBN 0-7099-1931-X
ISBN 0-7099-1938-7 (Pbk)

CONTENTS

Preface

Acknowledgements

To Lizzie and Jen

PREFACE

On first consideration the idea of a book on
violence for those in the caring professions may
appear anomalous. Those whose task it is to care
for others, we might imagine, would be the least
likely to encounter violent behaviour. In practice,
however, professionals may encounter a good deal of
hostility from those they are trying to help. That
psychiatric nurses, for example, encounter violence
may be unsurprising, but that general nurses do so
may be less obvious. Part of the problem is that
the kinds of problems which lead people to seek help
may also lead people to violent behaviour. Thus the
pain of an injury may increase irritability in an
individual presenting with such pain at a hospital,
or a drink problem may lead someone to seek help
simultaneously reducing their self-control. In a
number of ways the well-meaning and helpful
professional may have the problem of a clientele
whose propensity to violence is higher than normal.

Other factors also make violence a problem for
the helping professions. Increasingly social
workers, psychotherapists, psychiatrists and others
are being asked for help by violent individuals who
wish to change their own behaviour. To this may be
added the observation that many professions more
traditionally associated with the control of
violence are, with the adoption of a pastoral role,
becoming involved in its treatment. Thus such
groups as prison officers and police officers are
increasingly becoming involved in direct treatment
of problematic aggression.

Unfortunately the need for the involvement of
such professionals in the treatment of violence is
rarely matched by the availability of resources.
The lack of such resources became apparent to one of
us (G.O.) when involved in the planning of a course

on the "care of the violent and potentially violent individual". In particular the available reading material had a number of problems. Much was simply out of date, inevitable in any scientific field but a particular problem in the area of violence where knowledge is growing rapidly. More recent material, too, had its problems. Many texts provided only a hopelessly simplistic and impractical viewpoint; typically a textbook would give one particular theorist's viewpoint. Yet our understanding of violence has been greatly improved by workers in a number of different fields including anthropology, biology, psychology etc. To omit any of these is to give only a partial account of the problem.

Where texts from a multidisciplinary perspective did appear, all too often they turned out to be highly technical, obscure and unclear in their practical implications. Moreover their authors, writing largely for academics rather then workers in the field, all too often assumed a technical expertise which few "front-line" workers would possess.

The present book aims then to provide an up to date, readable and practical guide to the problem of violent behaviour. Inevitably keeping the book to a manageable size has necessitated the omission of a good deal of material. In general we have considered such issues as relevance, soundness and practical value in deciding what to include; in the final analysis however such decisions are our own personal ones and inevitably there will be some who disagree with our selection. One topic however, which we were convinced should be included, was the evaluation of work in violence, both as regards treatment and research. Since more and more information is constantly becoming available regarding violence it seems important that professionals should know how to evaluate it. This book therefore aims not only to give professionals a grounding in treatment and research on violence but also to equip them further to develop this knowledge in the future.

ACKNOWLEDGEMENTS

Many people have contributed directly or indirectly to the preparation of this book. Our particular thanks must go to Gerry Meenz and Dave Tully, formerly of Moss Side and Park Lane Hospitals, whose development of training courses on problems of violence provided much of the structure and purpose of the book and whose comments on early manuscripts were of great value. Our thanks also go to Di Brennand who so admirably typed the manuscript, Tim Hardwick who waited so patiently for it, and lastly to our patients, who taught us what to include in it.

Chapter One

THE HISTORICAL CONTEXT

If one thing is certain about human interaction, it is that violence between individuals and between groups of individuals is not new. Archaeological evidence shows that ever since the dawn of human history, human beings were dealing lethal blows to each other. Human remains attest to the fact that primitive people dealt death to their fellow human beings in as individually violent a way as their modern counterparts.

Moving from prehistory to the early days of recorded history, it becomes apparent that violence was an accepted part of the everyday life of the Roman citizen. Apart from the violence of incessant wars and subjugation of conquered peoples, we are told, by Pliny the younger, of the violence exhibited by the crowds of supporters at chariot races in the Circus Maximus. Fighting poured onto the streets of Rome and Constantinople and gangs of "fans" were able to "control" areas of the cities, in much the same ways as groups of football supporters hold on to territories on the terraces. The Roman games themselves evolved from sporting competition to scenes of ritualised killing varying in content from battles between armies of gladiators to orgies of torture and murder for the "entertainment" of the citizenry.

The recorded history of Britain and Europe in general is littered with examples of, in many cases, extreme violence, which on the face of it, at least, appeared to have no economic or political purpose. It has been argued that the codes of chivalry which evolved during the Middle Ages helped to bring the inherent violence of the relatively primitive European society under some sort of control. It was only when the sheer weight of numbers or when political or economic aims were overriding that the

1

constraints of chivalry were broken, and even here there is evidence that, at least among the higher strata of medieval society, military violence was influenced by chivalrous ritual. Ritual combat changed little throughout the Middle Ages, and even in the sixteenth and seventeenth centuries, it was fairly commonplace for participants to be killed. We are told that in France between 1589 and 1608, no less than eight thousand people were killed in sword fighting.

Violence as a means of settling disputes between individuals goes back well into antiquity. British history is in many ways the history of government, andthe history of English criminal, and to some extent civil, law is the story of the attempt by government to control the violence between individuals in cases of dispute. It is important to remember that the active and compelling part that the law plays in social relations today has not always been the case. Nowadays, the law is often enforced irrespective of the submission of the individual to its jurisdiction. If a "crime" is committed, the law is normally set in motion whether the injured party wishes it or not. This has certainly not always been so. In Anglo-Saxon England, for example, an injury done was primarily the affair of injured parties and their families. It was for them to avenge the wrong on the wrongdoer and the wrongdoer's family, and to prosecute a "blood feud" against them until the wrong was corrected by retaliation.

In quite early times, however, we find the leaders of society attempting to place restrictions on violence in the form of "blood feuds", by inducing the wrongdoer to offer compensation for the wrong done, and the injured party to accept this compensation. Tariffs of compensation (Bot) were promulgated, which attempted to redress the injury in terms of the extent of the wrong and the status of the sufferer. Moreover these compensations were not limited to disputes over property, but may in themselves be compensations for violent attacks. Thus we may see in the laws of King Alfred:"If the big toe be cut off let twenty shillings be paid to him as bot. If it be the second toe, fifteen shillings, if the middlemost toe, nine shillings. If the fourth toe, six shillings..." Nevertheless, the initiative of prosecuting and the power to compromise were still with the injured party; moreover if compensation was refused, the law had no means to enforce its payment. It was also the case that, even at this time, there were many offences for which compensation could not completely atone, but which also entailed a fine (Wite) payable to the king. What is more, and this is of some importance, there were crimes which were considered "botless" and which were punishable by death or mutilation and entailed a forfeiture of the offender's property to the king. The later Anglo-Saxon kings extended these "botless" offences, possibly for financial reasons, and hence in the laws of Canute it is laid down that the rights which the king enjoyed over all citizens of Wessex were: "Breach of the King's Peace, house-breaking, ambush, the receiving of outlaws and neglect of the summons to the army".

Today, we consider that any illegal violence is a "breach of the peace". However, the "King's Peace" of Canute did not have this extended meaning. It only extended to all places some of the time and to some places all of the time. For example, it covered the King's Household and his officers and the few great roads of England (the "King's Highway") at all times, and it applied to all places on the great festivals of the Church. However, there were many places and occasions in which an illegal act of violence did not break the "King's Peace" although it may break a lesser man's "peace". Every freeman had a "peace" of his own, which if breached constituted an offence varying in seriousness proportionate to the importance of its owner.

The coming of the Normans to England saw the establishment of a strong central monarchy. The King and central government ("Curia Regis") took over the administration of local justice by removing the local dignitaries from the administration of district justice and substituted the King's appointee, the sheriff. Whilst procedures remained much the same as before, the warrior-like traditions of the Normans, deriving as they did from the Vikings, allowed for trial by battle. At first this may not have been imposed upon the Anglo-Saxons, but in time, with the disappearance of the distinction between the two groups, trial by battle became a universal mode of trial. This method took its place alongside trial by the ordeals of fire or water. At the same time, trial by jury was becoming more used and developed from the establishment of the principle that localities were responsible for the maintenance of the King's Peace. The prime function of the jury was not to make judgement but to present and assess the evidence. A clearer distinction began to be made between "Pleas of the Crown", which were wrongs peculiarly within the cognizance of the Crown, and other offences. However, even until the end of the reign of Henry I (1100-1135), there was no general broad principle that acts of violence were royal pleas and entailed forfeiture to the Crown. Nevertheless, by the reign of Richard I(1189-1199), any act of violence, wherever and whenever committed, was a breach of the King's Peace and was punishable by the King's Judges. By the end of the twelfth century, all serious offences involving Breach of the Peace were heard in the royal courts. More serious offences placed "life and limb" in the King's hands and were subject to prosecution by the King.

By this time we can begin to distinguish between two types of crime: felony and misdemeanour. Whilst it has never been the case that this distinction referred merely to the nature of the criminal act, it is, on the whole, true that felony was the more serious. The real distinction, however, lay in the consequences, and it is here that we see the imposition of judicial violence. Conviction for felony meant death by hanging and loss of lands and chattels, whereas conviction for misdemeanour meant fine or short imprisonment.

As trial by ordeal fell into disrepute, a person charged with felony had to consent to trial by jury. Often, this consent would not be forthcoming and the accused would be kept in prison until such consent was obtained. Gradually the reason for this rule disappeared, and imprisonment became more and more rigorous and developed into the use of torture (the "peine forte et dure") designed to extract a submission to trial by jury. It was not until 1772 that a refusal to be tried by a jury in cases of felony was made equivalent to confession. Until then, if the accused died under torture whilst consent was being extracted for trial by jury, there was no conviction, and therefore land and chattels did not become forfeit. Trial by jury became therefore normal practice on indictment by suit of the King, although in private criminal appeals, the accused could in a normal case offer defence by battle. This procedure was not, however, open to women and indeed, if there was a violent presumption of guilt, the accused could be hanged immediately without trial.

In the thirteenth century, the initiative for criminal law passed to Parliament. In the next four

centuries, Parliament was mainly responsible for the
definition of new crimes and by the end of the
eighteenth century, the list of felonies had grown
from a dozen to over three hundred. It was no
longer possible to say that felonies were the more
serious crimes. What today would be regarded as the
relatively trivial offences of, say, wounding a
horse or making a false entry in a marriage
register, or even activities which nowadays would
not be seen as necessarily undesirable, such as
consorting with gypsies, were equally felonies with
murder and rape.

Loopholes in the law became common practice and
devices to allow for the full vigour of capital
punishment not to have to be applied for all
felonies were widespread. By the fifteenth century,
all people who could read could claim "benefit of
clergy", a device originally intended to ensure that
ecclesiastics, after conviction in the civil courts,
could be handed over to the Church for punishment.
On the other hand, Parliament began to patch up
these holes and by the beginning of the seventeenth
century, statutes had been established which allowed
for some of the so-called "clergyable" offences to
be punished by imprisonment or deportation. Until
well into the nineteenth century, the criminal law
had become antiquated and barbarous. In 1814, for
example, three boys, aged eight, nine and eleven,
were sentenced to death for stealing a pair of
shoes.

The great reforms of the nineteenth and
twentieth centuries generally worked to "humanise"
the application of the criminal law. This, together
with the influence of groups such as the Howard
League for Penal Reform, has kept the debate
concerning "Law and Order" in the political arena.

Modern media of communication have reflected
(some would say produced) an increased public
awareness of the application of law to the control
of crime, particularly violent crime, and since the
formation of a police force in the nineteenth
century, the control of crime in our society has
become a pervasive function of state.

It would be remiss not to consider the
historical context of violent behaviour in society
without considering that most extreme example of
organized violence, warfare. If social history is
to a large extent concerned with the development of
of government and law, political history is very
much concerned with war.

The development of the nation state in Europe

after the Romans was dependent on the emergence of organizations devoted to the promulgation of warfare. The feudal system was as much to do with the raising of fighting forces as it was to do with economic organization. The defence of territory against warring "barbarians" allowed, for example, the Church to accept, or indeed even to encourage, the prosecution of war; the codes of chivalry to which we have already alluded, took on the virtues of godliness, on the one hand to control the excesses within Christendom, but also to legitimize it against the Infidel, on the other.

As a piece of human social activity, warfare has had, and continues to have, an enormous amount spoken and written about it. There is an accepted difference between violence emitted between individuals and small groups, such as "gang fights", and wars, and this difference is as much to do with the scale and, certainly, in modern times, the all-pervasiveness of it, as it is to with national economic or ideological issues. As an example of the cause of human suffering, death and injury, warfare throughout history must be prime.

Warfare is normally studied in macro terms. We rarely analyse the significance of the behaviour of individual soldiers (though there are exceptions viz. Keegan,1976), but refer to the effect of "armies" and "battles". Individual violence is determined by the "state of war". Indeed, it may be argued that as warfare has developed through history, the technology of armaments has decreased the level of individual violence. What is violent about pushing a button to trigger off a nuclear bomb? It is difficult to conceptualise the scale of warfare and to compare wars on the basis of simple numbers. Richardson suggested that a logarithmic scale to show the number of deaths occurring in any one war was the most appropriate method of making comparisons. By this method, D(number of deaths) is represented by M(magnitude of war) in the formula $M=\log 10\ D$. On this scale the Boer War had 'a magnitude of 4.4 (25,120), the American Civil War, a magnitude of 5.8 (631,000) and the Second World War, a magnitude of 7.8 (25,000,000). The total destruction of the world would have a magnitude of approximately 9.4, the Falklands War 2.5 and the number of murders in Britain in a year 1.2. Perhaps this should serve to remind us that in terms of scale, violence IN society is miniscule compared to violence BY society.

PRACTICAL IMPLICATIONS

We may see then that although, at first, it may be
tempting to follow the remark attributed Henry Ford,
that "history is bunk", and therefore that
historical evidence regarding violence would have no
implications for our present-day problems, this is
not necessarily the case.

Some feel that, contrary to the above opinion, a
knowledge of a phenomenon's historical context is
essential to a full understanding. Certainly, it
does seem possible to note certain practical
implications of the information contained in the
present chapter. Among these are the following:

1. It is necessary to be cautious about describing
a form of violence as "new".
Violence is not a purely modern phenomenon, and even
the types of violence we encounter today have
remarkable parallels in history. This suggests that
any attempt to understand, for example, the violence
of the football "hooligan", must also look for
causes which would also have produced "chariot race
hooligans" in Ancient Rome (always remembering, of
course, that the parallels may be only superficial).
The notion that we live in an age of "unprecedented
violence" ignores periods of history which certainly
seem to have been more violent than our own.

2. Just as the FORM of violence may not be a purely
modern phenomenon, so the EXTENT of today's violence
is not necessarily without parallels. Violent crime
rarely produces a death rate comparable to that
reported as occurring due to duelling, in France, in
the sixteenth century. We should be wary,
therefore, of claiming that today is the most
violent period of history, and again, should be
cautious of attempts to attribute "rises" in
violence to purely modern causes.

3. Violence should not be seen as something which
occurs only illegally. Historically, violence has
occurred, and still does occur, within the law. Not
only has violence been a commonplace phenomenon
amongst criminal activities historically, so it has
been common in the judicial process. The use of
legal torture, still occurring in some form in many
"civilised" countries, provides an example which,
though apparently antithetical to our modern notions
of "freedom under the law" and "trial by our peers",
was a major method of implementing the judicial

system. The English legal system has hardly had a
history of being "soft" on offenders, but when its
activities were very brutal to convicted offenders,
there is no evidence that violent crime was ever
eliminated.

4. In terms of scale, violence IN society cannot
compete with the violence committed BY society in
the form of warfare.

Chapter Two

THE PRESENT PROBLEM

As we have seen in Chapter One much of English law has been concerned with the control of violence, often by producing a violent response itself. Obviously a large part of the violence in our society is illegal, though by no means all. Some violence is explicitly legitimised and condoned, perhaps the most obvious being the physical punishment of children by adults. In addition, besides the strictly illegal and the strictly legal there exist a number of 'grey areas' where for example violence may be technically illegal but where a judicial response is either absent or subordinate to other societal responses; violence within the family, in particular, will often fall into such a category.

Nevertheless it seems appropriate to begin a consideration of violence in modern society by examining criminal violence, the manifestation most commonly seen as important when the topic of violence is raised.

CRIMINAL VIOLENCE

In considering the incidence of particular crimes, or crime in general, in the United Kingdom the most important single source of information is probably the annual Home Office report on Criminal Statistics. Home Office statistics separate out the various recorded crimes into several categories. Most crimes of violence would be categorised as "serious offences" or indictable/triable either way offences and as such may be sub-categorised as "crimes against the person". These include murder, attempted murder, manslaughter, infanticide, wounding or other acts endangering life, as one might expect, but may also include "crimes against

the person". These include murder, attempted
murder, manslaughter, infanticide, wounding or other
acts endangering life, as one might expect, but may
also include "crimes against the person" which one
might not necessarily regard as violent such as
"procuring illegal abortion" or "concealment of
birth". Similarly another category of serious crime
would be "sexual offences", which may or may not
include crimes of violence, e.g. "rape", "indecent
assault on a female" but also "indecency between
males" and "bigamy". As one might expect, the
precise amount of criminal violence in society is
very difficult to estimate and the statistics
themselves, apart from the difficulties of inclusion
and exclusion as mentioned above, are also affected
by changes in the law and the use of court
proceedings.

About 2.5 million serious offences were recorded
in England and Wales for 1979. Of these, about 3.7%
were recorded as "violence against the person", and
0.9% were sexual offences. From 1969 to 1979
"violence against the person" offences rose by an
average of about 10% per year. Whilst there is a
clear tendency for the number of violent

1970	1971	1972	1973	1974	1975	1976	1977	1978	1979
8.7	14.4	11.5	17.0	4.1	11.3	9.4	5.8	6.0	9.1

All violence

4.7	11.1	4.0	9.6	5.3	3.3	-8.1	3.5	-1.6	1.7

Most serious

1969-1979; All violence: 151.3%; Most serious: 37.2%

offences to have increased over the last decade or
so, this trend is not so obvious for more serious
crimes of violence, and sexual offences actually
decreased in frequency during this period.

1970	1971	1972	1973	1974	1975	1976	1977	1978	1979
3.0	-2.5	-0.4	9.4	-3.9	-4.0	-6.3	-4.1	4.2	-2.7

1969-1979: -7.2%

Of all serious offences recorded, crimes of
violence and sexual offences are amongst those
having the highest "clear up" rate by the police
(about 80%). This may well contribute to the
impression that we live in a violent society, since

much of the popular reporting of crime comes from reports of cases brought to court. It should be remembered that violent crime accounts for a relatively small proportion of total serious crime and societal condemnation and sensitivity to it may increase the pressure on the police to clear up the reported crime and for members of society to report it. There is a reluctance to "sort out" problems informally, as in the past, possibly as a result of break up of extended families.

Use of Weapons

There is little doubt that the use of firearms in serious crime has increased substantially over the past decade or so. Of all offences involving firearms between 1969 and 1979, about a half were violence against the person offences, this representing about 3.4% of all such offences. However it is of considerable interest to note that the use of air guns, which are cheap and easily obtainable, went up by 757.2%, whereas the use of other, presumably more expensive and less easily obtainable weapons, went up by only 106.6% over the same period; moreover the proportion of crimes of violence against the person using weapons over other crimes using weapons reduced over the period (-17%).

1970	1971	1972	1973	1974	1975	1976	1977	1978	1979
6.8	31.0	20.0	27.9	3.3	28.0	16.9	-0.9	9.4	16.7

Violence against the person involving firearms:
% change over previous year

1970	1971	1972	1973	1974	1975	1976	1977	1978	1979
3.8	27.7	19.4	19.1	14.7	36.1	20.3	14.5	7.0	15.4

All serious offences using firearms
% change over previous year

1970	1971	1972	1973	1974	1975	1976	1977	1978	1979
13.5	32.3	43.6	28.8	13.2	33.9	27.4	15.8	15.4	19.6

Offences in which air gun was principal weapon
% change over previous year

1970	1971	1972	1973	1974	1975	1976	1977	1978	1979
-4.2	23.1	-6.0	3.6	17.6	40.5	7.3	11.6	-12.0	3.1

All other weapons: % change over previous year

Of course it is important to exercise a degree of caution in interpreting such figures. An increase in crime figures may be produced by a number of factors besides an actual increase in the amount of violence in society. Such factors may include changes in reporting practices by the general public and changes in the pattern of prosecutions. Thus changes in the structure of local communities may mean that the person who would once have dealt with a violence problem personally may now be more likely to involve the police. At one time, for example, an assault on a member of the family would, in many social groups, result in some other member of the family (a stronger elder brother for example) seeking out the offender and obtaining revenge directly. Changes in social practice may result in the same offence now appearing in the criminal statistics as a result of being reported to the police. Nevertheless it is clear that even allowing for such effects inflating the figures, criminal violence represents a substantial problem requiring an effective response on the part of society.

Societal Responses to Violent Crime.
For much of history, the state, particularly in developed societies, has sought to respond to crimes perpetrated by its members. As indicated earlier, these methods have included the death penalty, physical torture, social degradation (such as the ducking stool and the pillory), banishment and transportation, imprisonment and financial penalties.

Society's response to violent crime is, on conviction, to apply a system of sentences. Of those convicted in 1979 of serious offences (including violence against the person), one in ten received an immediate prison sentence and almost half were fined.

Sentencing
We can identify three types of justification for the legal response to crime.

The Present Problem

1. Retribution

This holds that the justification is that the offender deserves it because of the offence. It is usually "limited" to the extent that the punishment should not exceed what would match the offence; hence we have the statutory "maximum" sentences. Sentences are usually also "distributive" in the sense that culpability must be shown.

2. The Expressive or Denunciatory

This is the public expression of an important statement about the offence and is only just distinguishable from the utilitarian. It can also be argued that this justification (Walker 1980) requires a retributive element. For example, the use of suspended sentences can be regarded as declaring disapproval of an offence without the actual imposition of that sentence, but indicates how society would impose retribution were justice not being tempered by mercy.

3. Reductive or Utilitarian

This justification views sentencing as reducing the frequency of offences in one or more of the following ways:-

(a) deterrence of the offender, by the memory of the offender
(b) deterrence of imitators, by the publication of the sentence
(c) reformation of the offender, by education
(d) education of the public to take a more serious view of such offences
(e) protection of the public by the incapacitation of the offender

Clearly the first two of these three major categorisations of justification for sentencing are beyond the scope of this book and therefore our aim must be to examine some aspects of the utilitarian justification.

Deterrence of the Offender

The relevance of re-conviction rates here is obviously high and indeed there is little other evidence that might be used. The Home Office regularly publishes statistics on this. In 1977 for example the following statistics were obtained:

Principal Offence of conviction	Total	No previous convictions	1 or more
violence against the person.	46100	40%	60%
sexual offences.	8900	48%	52%

On the face of it, this would suggest that previous convictions and, presumably sentences, have not affected 60% and 52% of those convicted in 1977 of violence against the person or sexual offences. However, once again, one must exercise extreme caution in interpreting these figures. "Previous convictions" means convictions for any standard list offence other than a motoring offence and may not have been a violent or sexual offence. Also one cannot ascertain the extent to which a previous conviction would aid detection by the police. Hence if a person is known by the police to have committed a similar offence, that person may become a prima facie suspect.

Similarly if we consider reconviction rates after the imposition of varying length of prison sentences, we are really unable to determine effectiveness.

This can be illustrated clearly if we take an example. In 1976, of those receiving sentences of from three months to eighteen months' imprisonment, fifty-three per cent were reconvictions. Those receiving sentences of from eighteen months to four years, thirty-three per cent were reconvictions. Ostensibly, it would appear that the longer the prison sentence, the lower the reconviction rate. The problem here, of course, is that the this would not necessarily be the pure effect of sentencing but may reflect deterrence of the would-be offender, the type of crime and type of offender as much. In any event, the length of prison sentence per se would not appear to have an enormous effect.

Deterrence of the Would-be Offender.
Doubt about the deterrent effect on others of sentencing was seriously expressed over the application of the death penalty for murder. Clearly, capital punishment can be seen as having a deterrent effect only on would-be offenders, as it completely rules out the possibility of reoffending in the actual offender. Opponents of the death penalty look at the experience of various states in North America, the Commonwealth and Europe, where by

quasi-experiment, evidence would seem to show that the presence or absence of the death penalty is not related to conviction rates. In New Zealand, for example, where the death sentence has been repeatedly imposed and abolished, the murder rate does not seem to have been affected (Walker 1968, Sutherland and Cressy 1969). This does not, of course, mean that capital punishment is not a deterrent, but that in the context of alternative punishments, normally long prison sentences, the differential effect is minimal.

Reformation of the Offender.

Modern society officially regards the sentencing of criminals as serving basically a reformatory function. Most prisons and institutions for young offenders in Britain put great emphasis on the provision of facilities for educating and enlightening its inmates. Non custodial sentences may also reflect this aspect, with the use of "community service" sentences which, apart from having a restitutional or reparative function, may seek to educate the offender about the society to which he or she is obligated.

Education of the Public to take a Serious View of Offences.

Little is known about the effect of sentencing on public opinion about particular crimes. For one thing, it is uncertain which way the process flows in particular cases. For example, does the softening of public opinion towards such behaviour as homosexual activity between consenting adults show changes consequent upon the de-criminalisation of this behaviour, or conversely did the de-criminalisation follow the mood of public opinion? Some have maintained that the significant contribution of punishment is the legal sentiments, legal conscience, or moral feelings which have been developed in the general public by the administration of the criminal law over many generations which have become so organized that they regulate behaviour spontaneously.

Protection of the Public by the Incapacitation of the Offender.

Recent calls for the imposition of severe sentences for serious crimes undoubtedly contain an element of the urge to incapacitate the offender. It is certainly arguable that, for example, during custodial sentences the convicted criminal is unable to commit further crimes. Whether it makes sense, however, on these grounds is debatable, since this would have a substantial effect only on those crimes which were committed at a high frequency. As this does not normally apply to serious crimes, which by any one person typically occur only infrequently, a long custodial sentence may have little or no effect on inhibiting crime by incapacitation.

It can be seen, therefore, that criminal violence is a substantial problem in society; moreover it would appear that the efforts by society to deal with such violence are far from being entirely successful. Violence thus consititutes a problem for modern society even when seen only in terms of criminal violence: when we add to this the violence which does not primarily involve legal agencies it becomes clear that violence is appropriately a major cause for concern.

LEGITIMISED VIOLENCE

Not all violence in society is either illegal or proscribed. It is, for example, by no means uncommon to find that husbands consider themselves to have the right to physically assault their wives. Nevertheless, the law can be invoked, just as it can in the physical abuse of children. The law, however, is very uncertain about the use of violence in what is seen as corporal punishment. Parents are allowed to use physical punishment in the control of their children's behaviour, so long as this is not considered to be "excessive". Similarly, schoolteachers are given the right, when acting "in loco parentis" to inflict corporal punishment on their charges. Some idea of the extent of such violence can be obtained by close examination of school records.

In the United Kingdom schools are required by law to keep a punishment book in which all cases of corporal punishment are entered. Education Authorities, school inspectors, governors and managers have the right to scrutinize the punishment book. A study in 1974 showed that in Edinburgh during one term, more than 9500 cases were recorded of the the use of corporal punishment in the schools. Teachers themselves are divided on the use of corporal punishment in schools. One

organization, the Society of Teachers Opposed to
Physical Punishment, campaigns vigorously against
its use. Their argument rests mainly on the view
that it is an ineffective way of controlling
behaviour and creates an atmosphere in which it is
impossible to create good working relationships
between teacher and taught. They argue that use of
the cane teaches that, in the last resort, the way
to enforce one's will is by physical assault. Their
research suggests that even where teachers were
afraid of the abolition of corporal punishment,
their fears turned out to be unjustified when the
ban was effected. Until recently, parents could not
demand that corporal punishment was not inflicted on
their children in areas where no ban existed. If
they wished to protect their children from such
violence their only option was to move them to
schools where such a ban did exist. Britain, in
fact, has been slow to change this practice. All
eastern European and Common Market countries, except
Britain and Ireland, have abolished corporal
punishment in schools. Many of these countries
abolished it over a hundred years ago (Poland two
hundred years ago) and some countries also ban the
use of physical punishment in the home. After
European pressure, the British Government now allows
parents to opt out of the use of physical punishment
for their children in any school. Physical
punishment within the home is still permitted, with
little in the way of explicit guidelines regarding
how violent a parent may be before such punishment
be considered excessive. Indeed within the family a
considerable amount of violence may occur, with such
violence commonly being seen as legitimate and
normal. The recognition in recent years of the
amount of violence present in some families, with
the consequent risk to family members, makes it
appropriate to consider in detail the "grey area" of
social violence.

Social Violence
Falling somewhere between the violence which is seen
as clearly criminal (e.g. assault occasioning
grievous bodily harm, murder etc.) and that which is
seen as clearly legal (e.g. parental spanking of a
child - in most countries) fall a number of episodes
of violence which might reasonably be considered as
"social violence". Such violence, whilst not
strictly legal, does not simply result in the
occurrence of criminal charges. Either the violence

is dealt with within the social context of its
occurence, or external agencies (e.g. police, social
workers) are involved, but not primarily in order to
bring criminal charges. The most common of such
violence is perhaps that which occurs within the
family, particularly the forms of violence which
have come to be known as "the battered child" and
"the battered wife".

The "Battered Child"

From time to time the media produce horrified
accounts of episodes in which a small child has been
either badly injured, or even killed, by a violent
parent. Such physical abuse has come to be
described by professionals as "non-accidental
injury", a term generally preferred because (a) it
states more clearly what is the matter for concern -
people may disagree as to what actually counts as
"battering", but agree that there is an injury and
that the infliction was not accidental (b) much of
the subject matter of concern to professionals may
concern injuries not inflicted by physical beating,
but rather involving such injuries as burns or cuts
(c)"non accidental injury" is a somewhat less
emotive term, making it easier to consider the
details of each case calmly rather than in a state
of heated emotional outrage.

The incidence of non-accidental injury cases can
only be roughly estimated because of the
difficulties of detection associated with the
problem. However, in evidence to a select committee
of the House of Commons, the Royal College of
Psychiatrists has estimated that of children under
four years in England and Wales, 1 in 10,000 will
die as a result of physical abuse, and a further 9
will be severely injured. This is a high figure:
it implies that of all the children under four in
England and Wales, around 3,000 will be severely
injured each year, with 300 of those - six a week -
dying of their injuries. Such figures are easier to
estimate than those for moderate or mild cases: for
these a figure of 40-60/10,000 has been suggested.
Inevitably disagreement as to what constitutes child
abuse will lead to corresponding disagreement
regarding the size of the problem. Nevertheless it
is clear that the problem is serious and warrants
major concern.

It is of course important to note that child
abuse is not a new phenomenon. It is said (Kempe
and Kempe 1978) that 80% of illegitimate children

put out to nurse in 19th Century London died. Various forms of mutilation continue to this day for reasons of social custom or religious imperative. Nor is this a remote or distant problem: female circumcision (surgical removal of the clitoris) has recently become a matter of concern in the United Kingdom, with Parliament discussing the possible need for legislation for its control. The formal recognition of child abuse is however a relatively recent phonomenon, and it was not until 1962 that the Journal of the American Medical Association reported on a meeting of the American Academy of Paediatricians on "the battered-child syndrome". Since then information, research and legislation has mushroomed and public awareness of the problem has done much to reduce the size of the problem: Kempe and Kempe (1978) for example report that in Denver the number of hospitalised children dying from their injuries has dropped from 20 per year to less than one per year between 1960 and 1975. The most important factor in this reduction appears to be that cases are milder, suggesting that families are being helped sooner.

The Appearance of the Problem

The clinical features of the abused child have been outlined by Hull (1974), who describes bruising, bony injuries and head injuries. In all of these there are some difficulties in distinguishing, in toddlers, accidental and non-accidental injury. Bruises due to accident are common on forehead and legs in toddlers. In an immobile baby accidental bruising is rare, and in all babies bruising around mouth, chest or abdomen are all suspicious signs. Fractures, like bruises, are unlikely in immobile babies, and complete (rather than greenstick) fractures are rare in toddlers. Commonly the factors associated with non-accidental injury relate to the fact that the bone is not yet fully developed; Hull notes that swinging a baby by a limb can produce two clear X-ray findings, epiphysial separation (separation of the growing part of the bone from the existing long bone) and periosteal thickening (produced by squeezing of the limb where the bone is surrounded by a thin envelope, the periosteum).

Head injuries present a greater diagnostic problem in that both fractures and subdural haematomas (bleeding around the brain) may occur for a variety of reasons (e.g. accidental dropping). On

19

the other hand such injuries may reflect the squeezing of the baby by the arm or leg such that their skulls strike a hard surface, or in the case of sub-dural haematoma, the result of vigorous shaking causing rupture of delicate blood vessels around the brain. Thus in one case of the first author's, a four month old baby suffered a fractured skull on being thrown violently back into his cot after his mother had failed to stop him crying.

It should be noted, however, that a large number of other injuries may be sustained by the victims of child abuse. Such injuries may include rupture of internal organs, evidence of violent insertion of instruments to the child's mouth or rectum, burns or tooth marks: Lee (1978) for example describes injuries in which part of a child's testicle was removed by a bite from the mother.

Research into Non-accidental Injury

Besides straightforward research into the incidence, types and severity of injuries, much research has been conducted into the origins of non-accidental injury. Such research has generally concentrated on characteristics of parents, children, or their relationship and the evaluation of therapeutic strategies.

Characteristics of the Abusing Parent

In general few consistent findings are available regarding the characteristics of abusing parents. Abusing mothers have generally been described as of lower age than average, even when allowance is made for the effects of social class (Smith 1975). It has popularly been reported that abusing mothers were themselves typically abused children: whilst there is evidence to support this notion (e.g. Oliver 1974) it is important to remember that much of this research depends upon the distant memories of parents in what will typically be a stressful situation. Moreover such studies commonly involve a number of confounding variables, making it unclear to what extent the relationship is causal and to what extent merely correlational (Newberger and Daniel 1976, DeMause 1975). Parents have often been reported as coming predominantly from the lower social classes, although Kempe (1969) suggests that all social classes are represented in child abuse. Psychological findings are typically inconsistent: whilst "abnormality of personality" is a common

finding (e.g. Smith, 1975) such judgements are often
the subjective opinions of involved professionals
observing the parents in what is normally a
difficult situation. Consequently opinions may vary
dramatically: Smith (1975) reports 33.3% of fathers
psychopathic, in contrast with Kempe's (1969) report
of only 2-3%. Gil (1968) argued for the involvement
of alcoholism, but no such association was found by
Smith (1975). Such differences reflect in part the
methodological difficulties of the area, and in
particular problems associated with the definition
of abuse. Sometimes these problems may result from
administrative and political issues. Thus a
district with hard pressed social services may be
physically unable to cope with all the cases which
might constitute child abuse, and thus be forced to
restrict itself to the most severe or obvious forms.
Another, less hard pressed, district may be willing
to consider as child abuse a much wider variety of
forms. Researchers in the two areas, even if both
operating from the non-accidental injury register,
would then receive quite different pictures of child
abuse.

Characteristics of Children

Inevitably a similar problem occurs when considering
the characteristics of abused children, and here,
again, research can give quite variable results.
Thus the N.S.P.C.C. research team in their report
(1976) highlighted such factors as abnormality of
delivery, whether or not the child was wanted, and
whether or not the child presented problems (e.g.
sleeping, feeding problems) during the first three
months of life. Such variables are difficult to
interpret however: as the N.S.P.C.C. research team
point out, a mother's recollection of whether a
child produces problems may not be an entirely
reliable source of information. Thus Gregg and
Elmer (1969) reported that their assessments of the
characteristics of abused children showed them to be
no different from others: their mothers however
tended to remember them as having presented
problems. Even if the children do present greater
difficulties than others, it is difficult to know
how much of this is the cause of the parents'
hostility, and how much is a consequence.
Additionally there is the problem of seizing
upon certain variables, not because they are
suggested by the evidence, but because they seem
plausible. Thus in one case referred to the first

author the abused child had been, according to the
N.S.P.C.C. report, a forceps delivery, to a young
mother. To seize on these as causal factors would
be premature: the same mother had another
non-abused child, born some four years earlier, by
Caesarian delivery. Young age and difficult
delivery could not therefore, by themselves, be used
to provide an adequate explanation.

Characteristics of Parent Child Interaction

A number of studies have looked at characteristics
of the Parent-Child relationships and interactions
in the hope of adding to our understanding of
non-accidental injury. In particular a number of
workers have commented on the tendency of abusing
parents to make demands of their children which are
unrealistically high, both in terms of total demands
and the expectancy of what is appropriate to various
ages. Thus a child only a few months of age may be
seen by a parent as "wilfully" wetting a clean nappy
in order to irritate the mother who has just
replaced it. (See e.g. Kempe 1971, Steele and
Pollock 1968). They may thus see the child as
deliberately trying to make life difficult.
Resentment therefore ensues, with subsequent abuse.
   This pattern of interaction, in which demands
seem to be placed on the child to satisfy parental
needs for achievement, success etc., has been
described by a number of workers as "role reversal".
To some extent this appears to relate to the
commonly reported observation that abusing parents
themselves have unhappy, distorted, emotionally
deprived childhoods. The suggestion is that the
parent seeks from the child the reassurance and
success that they failed to experience as chldren.
As a causal explanation, however, such a notion
remains highly speculative.
   Various writers have suggested that a major
feature of the parents relationship to the abused
child is a "failure of bonding". The process of
"attachment", whereby bonding of the child to the
parent typically occurs, has been widely described
and documented (e.g. Bowlby 1958). Failure of such
bonding, it is argued, may be responsible for the
difficulty experienced by the abusing parent, both
in relating to the child and in controlling
aggressive impulses towards the child. Amongst the
factors thought to contribute to bonding
difficulties are parental illness, difficulty or
prematurity of pregnancy and delivery, whether the

pregnancy was planned and so on. Thus Ounsted et al. (1974) reported a number of physical and psychological problems in most of their parents of abused children, such problems being seen as contributory to failure of parent-child bonding.

As with most areas of research into child abuse, however, it is important to remember the methodological difficulties involved. In particular many studies do not provide adequate comparison data on interactions in non-abusing families. Such problems as the possible over-representation of lower social classes in child abuse inevitably lead to the risk that the higher social class professionals dealing with the problem will identify features of child rearing as indicative of risk factors, when they represent nothing more than, say, a social class difference. Much more confidence in the research would be possible if the abusing families could be directly compared with other non-abusing families, similar in as many respects as possible. Such a "control" group, strengthening the case for involvement of whatever factors are found to differ in the two groups, is often lacking in child abuse research; until studies with adequate controls are performed, it will remain difficult to draw conclusions on such issues as whether or not abused children do in fact become abusing parents.

Treatment in Child Abuse Cases
A number of strategies have been adopted by professionals dealing with child abuse cases. Inevitably recognition and labelling of an incident as "child abuse" or "non-accidental injury" results in the involvement of a good deal of legal and administrative machinery to do with the police, courts, social services and so on. At various points in these procedures it is necessary to develop suitable approaches to the treatment of abusing families.

The forms of such treatment vary considerably. In some cases parent and child may both be admitted to special units, perhaps in a group of other similar parents and children (see e.g. Ounsted et al. 1974). Other workers have concentrated on behavioural approaches to treatment, modelling appropriate interactions with the child, teaching self-control skills, setting formal goals and so on. Kempe and Helfer (1972) describe the use of "Parent Aides", lay workers who become involved with problem families on a medium to long-term basis.

Effectiveness of treatment procedures is however difficult to evaluate. Where evaluation has been done, results have often been encouraging but far from completely satisfactory. Thus although the N.S.P.C.C. Battered Child Research Team noted a number of improvements in the families in their study (1976) with "a diminished possibility of serious injury to most of the children" they added that "in only a few cases did we feel sufficiently confident to state that the risk of injury...was eliminated" (page 178). In a five-year follow up on non-accidental injury cases, Friedman and Morse (1976) obtained equivocal results, with formerly abused children requiring more hospital treatment for subsequent injuries, but not to an extent that was statistically significant.

Nevertheless, as mentioned earlier, there are reasons to believe that the various steps taken to deal with child abuse are helping to alleviate the problem. Hopefully further research will lead, if not to its total elimination, at least to a marked reduction.

The Battered Wife

Just as the term "battered baby"can be misleading, so can the term "battered wife", and for similar reasons: as yet, however, no satisfactory alternative term has come into general usage. Certainly violence of this nature is not uncommon: thus in one survey of 1,500 divorce complaints in Southern England, around 90% involved women who suffered "repeated violence in marriage" (Chester and Streather 1972). The Select Committee on Violence in Marriage (1975) recommended that refuge provision should be made for one in 10,000 of the population, implying a figure of 5 - 6,000 for the number of women in the United Kingdom needing such provision. Binney et al. (1981) however quote the Citizen's Advice Bureau as estimating dealing with 25,000 battered women per year. Inevitably a number of women who are subject to physical abuse do not come to the notice of the authorities, making it difficult to obtain figures which do not underestimate. Nevertheless, as with non-accidental injury to children, the problem is obviously severe.

Particularly striking in the area of battered wives, however, is the reported inadequacy of police action in dealing with the problem. Research on women in refuges in England and Wales has revealed that over 60% did not find the police useful (Pahl 1978, Binney et al. 1981). Whilst this figure inevitably reflects to some extent the nature of the sample (in that those who did find the police useful might not have needed the refuge), this still represents a disturbing number of women. In a detailed study of 59 women who had called the police, Binney et. al. (1981) found that 30 had had the assault described as a 'domestic dispute', with no practical help being given, and a further five reported that the police had not actually appeared. Whilst this may to some extent reflect the difficulty of bringing a strong enough case to court, other suggested reasons for failure to prosecute include the belief amongst police officers that power of arrest in family disputes should only be used as a last resort, discouragement by officers when women may wish to pursue a complaint, and the belief amongst officers that women will later withdraw the charges before the case. This latter belief, incidentally, seems to have little justification, research generally suggesting that only 5 - 10% of women in fact do withdraw charges (Binney et al. 1981).

The Appearance of the Problem

A number of writers have commented on the types of injury or abuse involved in wife-beating. Pizzey (1978) describes a number of cases involving broken bones, dislocations, bruising and so forth. Of 25 cases involving life threatening attacks, Binney et al. noted only five prosecutions: it appears therefore that the low level of prosecution does not reflect a low intensity of attack. Threats to life and limb are commonly reported, together with more bizarre forms of abuse: one of Binney et al.'s respondents reported being submerged in a cold water bath by her husband after he had lost money gambling. One study which broke down the forms of abuse into types was that of Dobash and Dobash (1980). They found punching to the face or body to account for almost half the attacks, kicking with butting or striking with the knee over a quarter of the remainder. Hitting with objects accounted for 5%, attempted smothering or strangling a further 2%. In addition many women report various forms of mental cruelty, including extreme dominance or use of threats. The use of verbal torments and threats resulted in many women becoming doubtful of their own sanity.

25

In general studies have found that violence
tends to begin, for most women, only after marriage:
again this may be unsurprising to the extent that
women are less likely to marry a man they already
know to be violent. Where violence started outside
marriage this was often after the women had started
to live with the man. It is possible therefore that
men may be more likely to be violent once they feel
they are in a powerful position and that escape
would be difficult for the women. For many women,
violence had continued for a long time before the
women found a means of escape, usually at a refuge.
Of the women in Binney et al's study (1981), a
quarter had suffered for ten years or more.

The observation that many women tolerate such
abuse for extended periods has given rise to the
notion that women who are victims of violence in
some way enjoy it, either consciously or
subconsciously. This notion has been further
encouraged by the observation that a number of women
return to violent partners, although Binney et al.
(1981) in their follow-up study, found that almost
90% of women in their sample were still apart from
their attacker 18 months later. Of the women who
had returned, around half had done so because of the
stress of being away, including threats and further
violence from their partner (one man burned down his
wife's new flat), wishing to regain children and so
on. Overall, women who had returned reported only
slight improvements in the relationship and that
they would like to leave again if they could find
somewhere suitable.

The notion that battered women are "asking for
it" seems to be less widely held than in the past,
particularly amongst those who are involved with
such work on a day-to-day basis: where such a
perspective is revived it is usually from those
whose involvement in the area is slight or who have
been involved but lost contact with the day-to-day
activities of care agencies. Thus Erin Pizzey, in
her 1978 reprinting of "Scream Quietly or the
Neighbours Will Hear" argued (page 37) that, in
response to the reaction 'a lot of them like it',
she had never met anyone who experienced this kind
of violence and wanted to stay with it. Soon
afterwards she left direct involvement in care of
battered women, spending several years in touring,
lecturing etc. Since then she has found herself
susceptible to the notion that women could enjoy
this kind of abuse, writing a book with her new
husband in which such a notion is proposed (Pizzey &

Shapiro 1982). Despite an illusion of scientific respectability, however, the work contains few facts, many opinions, and considerable discrepancy between the facts presented and the conclusions drawn. Much of the 'evidence' consists of anecdote or of accounts of, for example, interviews in which leading questions are common and in which the interviewer contradicts the interviewee (often a child) until the correct answer is given. Confident reference is made to studies of the relationships between hormones and behaviour, despite the problems of such studies (see Chapter Three). The impression is therefore of a theory with an initial plausibility but little if any factual support.

Systematic research on the reasons why women return to violent partners were collected by Binney et al. (1981). Amongst the reasons given, almost 60% of their sample reported problems with accommodation. Other reasons included being forced to return, returning for the sake of the children, and giving the partner another chance. One battered wife told the first author that she had returned to a violent husband several times, mainly because of the difficulty of finding somewhere else, partly because of self-doubts about it being in some way her own fault. On finding a refuge, she left for good. Disturbingly she commented that, had she read a book which appeared, scientifically, to show that victims 'asked for it' her mental state at the time would not have permitted her to doubt it. She would, she felt, have assumed that it must be true, and resigned herself to her fate.

Help for Battered Wives
Whilst various legal and social agencies have taken steps to provide help and support for the battered wife, it is probably fair to say that the biggest single source of help comes from the presence of refuges. Many areas now have accommodation available for women to escape from violent relationships, although these are often sparsely equipped, overcrowded and uncomfortable.

Binney et al. (1981) in their survey of refuge provision in the United Kingdom found that none of Britain's Metropolitan Districts had levels of refuge provision approaching that recommended by the Select Committee on Violence in Marriage. The highest provision was 60% of that recommended (W. Yorkshire), the lowest less than 6% (W. Midlands). The types of property varied enormously from large,

renovated detached houses to "short life" small
terraced houses in need of repair. Overcrowding was
commonly found, with some fifteen to twenty people
occupying a single house. Forty three per cent of
women had to share their bedroom with other
families. In general refuges have avoided refusing
entry to further women, despite overcrowding, since
the women concerned are aware not only of the
problems confronting other battered women but also
of the risk that a woman turned away may be
discouraged from seeking help again. It is not
unusual for refuges to be broken into by aggrieved
husbands, either to further harass their partner, or
even to direct hostility at other inhabitants after
their partner had left. Besides the personal
distress caused by such incidents, the ensuing
damage may introduce a further strain on the
refuge's limited finances. Whilst attempts are
typically made to keep the addresses of refuges
secret, such attempts are inevitably limited. Often
the woman's address is revealed during legal
proceedings. Many husbands show considerable
persistence and ingenuity in tracing their partners,
by such means as following their children home from
school, persuading well-meaning women to find the
refuge by pretending to be in distress, or simply by
walking the streets in likely areas until either the
partner or the children were seen.

On the positive side, however, the experience of
women in refuges has been such that they felt safe.
Around 80% of the women in Binney et al.'s (1981)
study reported feeling safe, and three quarters said
they had found the police useful in protecting the
refuge (far more than had found the police helpful
in protecting the marital home). Organisation of
refuges on a national basis through the Women's Aid
Federation provides a structure whereby help can be
found for women in other cities, enabling them to
move well away from their husbands.

Despite their problems it seems clear that
refuges provide a valuable service, possibly the
only really useful service in dealing with domestic
violence. Women continue to fill refuges to
capacity and beyond. Commonly the physical
protection is supplemented by help regarding such
issues as social security, rehousing etc. In
addition many women seem to welcome the opportunity
to share their experiences with other women.
Reactions of shame and embarrassment are commonplace
amongst victims of violence, and the opportunity to
talk to other victims has been seen as a valuable

part of restoring the woman's self-confidence. For all their limitations refuges have an essential part to play in dealing with a major social problem.

PRACTICAL IMPLICATIONS

Clearly the degree to which violence presents a problem in society is hard to determine precisely; nevertheless the evidence is sufficient to show that it is widespread. Amongst the points we may note regarding violence in society are the following:

1. Whilst the criminal statistics indicate general trends in violence, it is important to treat them with some degree of caution. In particular "offences against the person" is not synonymous with "violent offences". Similarly offences involving firearms may largely reflect the use of such weapons as airguns.

2. Much violence does not reach the criminal statistics or is not primarily the concern of legal agencies. In particular much, perhaps most, violence occurs within families, with the law either playing a minor role relative to such agencies as Social Services, or with no role at all in such instances as "normal" parental punishment of children.

3. In dealing with violent crime in society, judicial processes have failed to provide anything like an adequate solution. Social violence appears to be responding to measures introduced (e.g. refuges for wives, treatment for abusing parents) but here again much remains to be done. Much violence continues, particularly in the home and school, perpetuating the notion that violence in some circumstances is acceptable.

Chapter Three

THE BIOLOGICAL PERSPECTIVE

The influence of biology on theories of aggression
has been twofold. Besides the direct investigation
of physical processes in the determination of
behaviour, biology has also developed its own
approach to the study of behaviour, known as
ethology. The essence of ethology is the study of
behaviour in its natural setting. Ethological
studies have contributed greatly to our
understanding of aggression and violence in both
human and animal societies. Before considering this
particular perspective, however, it is appropriate
to look at some of the ways in which physical, as
well as behavioural, biology has added to the
understanding of aggressive behaviour.

1.   Hormonal Influences
A great deal of biological research on aggression
has been concerned with identifying ways in which
such behaviour may be affected by the body's hormone
levels. This research has centred mainly around the
influence of male sex hormones or androgens,
although other hormones have also been studied. In
one of the earliest experiments it was found that
castrated rats showed a lower level of aggression
than rats which have not been castrated. Further,
when the rats were given injections of the male sex
hormone testosterone their aggression levels rose to
those of other, non-castrated, rats. Similar
results have been reported for a number of different
species. Further support for the implication of
androgens comes from the observation that
testosterone levels in monkeys are correlated with
behavioural measures of aggressiveness: in general,
the higher the monkey's testosterone level, the
higher its level of aggressiveness (Rose et al.

1971). Studies also exist of human subjects. Doering et al. (1974) studied variations over time in serum testosterone levels of a group of men. The men were also asked to complete a series of ratings on such matters as how hostile they felt, how depressed and so on. Originally a weak correlation was reported between testosterone level and hostility, but in a later paper (1975) Doering and his colleagues suggested that this was not reliable: moreover it appeared that the level of testosterone correlated more highly with reports of depression than of hostility. It thus appears that the work on rodents may not relate in any straightforward way to human beings. Indeed other studies suggest that the effect may depend quite closely on the type of animal chosen for study: Morgan (1975) for example reported that the castration experiment, when repeated with dogs, failed to produce a lessening of aggressiveness. Even the research on dominance in monkeys is unclear. Thus Rose et al. (1972) paired two monkeys low in dominance with two other female monkeys whom they could dominate. The testosterone levels of the monkeys rose dramatically, suggesting that it was the domination which caused the high hormone level, rather than vice versa. Moreover, when the monkeys were returned, with their new high testosterone level, to a social group in which their ranking was low, their testosterone levels fell accordingly.

This is not to say, however, that hormones play no part in human aggression, but merely that we should be cautious about drawing conclusions too rapidly from animal research. Some human research still hints at a role for testosterone in the understanding of aggression. For example in one study (Yasoon et al. 1973) 20 sons of diabetic mothers were found by age 10 to show significantly less aggression than a control group. The importance of this study is that the mothers of the boys concerned had been given progesterone and oestrogen during pregnancy. As a result, it was suggested, the boys' brains had in some way been 'feminised', leading to lower aggression.

In understanding the role of testosterone in aggression two possible ways have been suggested in which it may operate. Firstly testosterone is considered to be possibly important in the development of the brain, sensitising it so as to enable it to detect testosterone later in life. Secondly it is believed that testosterone may need to be present in order for aggressive behaviour to be exhibited in certain situations. These two are of course not incompatible, and both could in fact be true, although as mentioned above the evidence regarding the role of androgens in human aggression is still far from clear.

Other hormones have of course been suggested as possibly playing a role in aggression. Experiments have suggested a reduction in aggression with chronic administration of addreno-corticotrophic hormone (ACTH), and an increase with acute administration of corticosterone. Such research studies however commonly suffer from the same problems mentioned above regarding androgens, and the picture is still far from clear. It seems that hormones and aggressive behaviour are capable of affecting each other, but it is still too soon to make any definite statements about the exact nature of such interrelationships.

2.   Genetic Factors

A second physical factor to have been implicated in aggression is the individual's genetic make-up. Again two possible ways have been suggested as to how this may happen. Firstly it is suggested that certain abnormal chromosome patterns may affect aggressive behaviour, some patterns increasing and others decreasing aggression. Secondly it is suggested that certain personality types, having at least some genetic basis, may be associated with aggressiveness. This latter possibility of course coincides with the general area of personality factors, and will not be discussed here but deferred to the section on personality factors in Chapter five.

Chromosome abnormality is a relatively recent field of study within medicine. Often relying on the use of high-magnification (electron) microscopy, it could not substantially develop until the technology became available in the 1950's.

The problems themselves are not particularly common: sex chromosome abnormalities for example have been reported as occurring with an incidence of around once per thousand births, the occurrence of an extra X chromosome possibly being slightly more common than the occurrence of an extra Y chromosome. Some chromosome abnormalities are rather more common, for example trisomy 21, a chromosome abnormality accounting for around 95% of cases of Down's syndrome (Mongolism) has been reported at around 1 in 1000 births, or as high as 1 in 200

births to mothers aged 35 or over. The occurence of
such types of abnormality has occasionally been
linked with aggressiveness, and because of this it
is useful to consider some of these abnormalities
more closely: not only is it then possible to learn
about aspects of aggressiveness specific to these
individuals, but also perhaps to learn a little
about how genetic factors in general may relate to
aggression.

Down's syndrome is now known to result from the
occurrence of an extra chromosome in the zygote
(fertilised egg). All the body's cells, developing
as they do from this original cell, contain a
corresponding extra chromosome, usually the
chromosome specified as No. 21, although less
commonly a different chromosome may be the extra
one.

Down's syndrome is characterised by a particular
type of physical structure including the "slanting"
eyes giving a mongoloid appearance (hence the early
name of the syndrome). In addition Down's syndrome
children are characterised by a degree of mental
handicap and, commonly, an increased susceptibility
to disease. Of interest in the present context,
victims of Down's syndrome have also been reported
to be characterised by lack of aggressiveness.

In practice it is not easy to show for certain
that victims of Down's syndrome are in fact less
aggressive than other individuals. Down's syndrome
victims differ in many ways from other people, and
it may simply be that one of these consequences of
Down's syndrome, rather than the syndrome itself,
leads to a reduced likelihood of aggression. For
example, it could be that the distinctive appearance
of the Down's syndrome child elicits more sympathy
from others, resulting in their being treated more
kindly and hence with less need for aggression.

Nevertheless there is at least some evidence in
support of the notion that aggressiveness is, on
average, lower in Down's syndrome victims than
others. Various studies have suggested that such
individuals tend to be described as more
affectionate, contented and cheerful than controls,
and one study reported that only 2 out of 38 were
hospitalised, by comparison with 26 out of 65 of a
similar non-Down's syndrome control group. One
interpretation of the latter is that the Down's
syndrome children may be more manageable, in
accordance with a hypothesis of lowered
aggressiveness.

On the other hand it must not be supposed that

Down's syndrome victims can never be aggressive. Down's syndrome victims have on a number of occasions been commited for treatment in secure mental hospitals, their level of violence being too great to enable them to remain in the community.

Thus, whilst many or most Down's syndrome victims may be less aggressive than other people, this will not necessarily be the case for all such individuals. Nevertheless the evidence does seem to give some support to a possible link between genetic abnormalities and some aggressive behaviour.

A second well-known type of chromosome abnormality affects the sex chromosomes in such a way that the individual has an extra 'Y' chromosome. This is the chromosome which, in the normal individual, determines that the individual will develop as a male rather than a female. In the male the chromosomes, instead of forming 23 matching pairs, consist of 22 matched pairs plus an asymmetric pair, the XY pair. The female on the other hand has two 'X' chromosomes, giving 23 symmetric pairs.

In the so-called XYY syndrome the individual has, instead of 46 chromosomes, a total of 47, resulting from the addition of an extra 'Y' chromosome. As mentioned earlier, such an abnormality is rare, occurring roughly once in every 1,000 births.

Individuals with the XYY syndrome are male, and have been described as having, on an average, greater height than normal males. Individually however they show no distinguishing physical characteristics.

Following studies of the sex chromosome characteristics of patients in secure mental hospitals it became apparent that such patients were much more·likely to be XYY patients than would be expected on the basis of the frequency of XYY in the normal population. The figures vary somewhat, but are clearly raised and of the order of thirty times the frequency in the normal population. That is to say, a male selected at random from the special hospitals is around 30 times as likely to be XYY as one selected from the population at large. On the other hand it should be noted that even such a disproportionate percentage still leaves only a small fraction of such patients showing chromosomal abnormality. Most patients in such institutions are of completely normal chromosomal makeup.

Nevertheless some workers have on the basis of this attempted to link such abnormalities with violent behaviour, a higher likelihood of antisocial behaviour amongst XYY males. Mark and Erwin (1970) for example, in their book "Violence and the Brain", call for more detailed studies of the behavioural implications of such abnormalities.

Detailed studies, however, of the records of detained XYY patients reveals that their offences are more likely to be property offences than offences against other people (see e.g. Casey et al. 1973). In a survey of XYY males admitted to United Kingdom Special Hospitals, Price (1978) noted that not only were the XYY men more likely to offend against property than people, but that the converse was true for corresponding XY patients. Moreover there is some evidence to suggest that only certain types of institution contain such disproportionate numbers of XYY individuals. Thus Jacobs et al. (1971), after screening 1,119 boys in approved schools, found a proportion not significantly different from the general population. Thus XYY men are not over-represented in all delinquent groups, and possibly only over-represented in those with psychiatric involvement. Moreover, even such men are, if anything, less likely to offend against other people than their peers. Finally it should be noted that even the number found in secure environments still account for only a small percentage of the XYY males in the population as a whole. By far the greatest majority of XYY men never come to the attention of the legal system at all.

Of course genetics may play a part in the production of aggressive behaviour without involving gross chromosomal abnormalities like XYY or Down's syndrome. Animal breeders have for many years been aware that they can breed docility or aggressiveness into an animal. Thus working animals like guard dogs or cattle may be selectively bred to encourage, respectively, ferocity or docility. In the same way many workers have speculated on the possibility that aggressiveness in humans may be, at least in part, genetically determined.

Early attempts to show genetic bases for a number of psychological problems gave results which seemed remarkably encouraging. Kallman, in a series of studies on schizophrenia, obtained data suggesting a concordance rate of 69% for monozygotic (identical) twins with only 11% for dizygotic (non-identical) twins. This, it was argued, reflected the greater genetic similarity of the former (see e.g. Kallman 1938). Other studies however have failed to provide support for such claims. Tienari (1963) for example reported figures consistent with a concordance figure of only 6% for monozygotic twins and 5% for dizygotic twins, a difference which could easily be accounted for by increased similarity of experience of twins of identical appearance.

A similar history of results is apparent when we turn to criminal behaviour. Thus Lange (1929) found 10 out of 13 monozygotic twins concordant by comparison with only 2 out of 17 dizygotic, leading him to a belief in substantial genetic determination of criminality. Similar belief in the genetic basis of criminal behaviour can be seen in many subsequent theories (see e.g. Eysenck 1964) as discussed in Chapter Five. Again, however, early work has not always been supported by the later, more carefully controlled studies. Thus Stampfl (1936) and Kreuz (1936) produced data suggesting 63% and 48% concordance between monozygotic and dizygotic pairs, results which again may reflect little more than increased similarity of treatment of physically similar individuals and which at least one worker in the field has described as "not very striking" (Shields 1973 p. 573).

In interpreting genetic studies a number of problems are apparent. Even the best of such studies need to be regarded with caution (see Chapter Eleven). Many of the studies, particularly the earlier ones, appear to be rather poorly conducted. In one of the early schizophrenia studies, for example, a third of the relatives were dead at the time the data was collected. A number of factors may serve to bias the results, including the increased similarity of treatment of twins of identical appearance by parents and peers. Specific estimates of genetic contribution may depend on a number of factors including the environmental conditions of the study (if the environments are similar, the proportion of variability due to genetics will be inflated), duration of exposure to the environment, age etc. Thus a behaviour may have a high genetic component under one set of conditions and only a low genetic component under others. As a result it is often difficult to do more than acknowledge that genetic factors are involved to some extent; whether they account for over 90% of the variation or less than 10% may depend on a large number of unspecified and even unknown circumstances. Since one's genetic make-up cannot be changed, any conclusion may be of limited practical value requiring at least a knowledge of the mechanism whereby the genetic factors operate. Such knowlege is obviously far from being available as yet, and studies of heritability are unlikely to contribute substantially to solving problems of violence in the near future.

3.   Neurological Factors

A third link between biology and aggression has come from research into neurological aspects of aggression. Such work has two quite distinct roots. On the one hand a large body of evidence from clinical sources suggests links between neurological disturbance and aggression. In addition a considerable body of experimental work has pointed to possible associations between the nervous system and aggression.

Experimental work has been dominated by two complementary approaches to the study of neurological structure. The first, known as electrical stimulation of the brain (ESB), involves the stimulation of specific parts of the brain in order to observe the behavioural consequences. Usually (but not always) this involves the more or less permanent insertion of electrodes into the region of interest.

The second approach, generally known as brain lesion studies, involves the isolation, by cutting or occasionally by removal, of specific brain structures. Their functions can then be identified by noting any subsequent behavioural loss or disruption.

Of the various studies which have attempted to investigate neural mechanisms implicated in aggression, perhaps the most dramatic have been those involving the electrical stimulation of the brain (ESB). In such experiments, microelectrodes are inserted into specific areas of the brains of experimental animals. Such areas can then be precisely stimulated providing clues as to their role in the whole brain system.

Although early work, during the 1920's and 1930's, was necessarily crude, even then it was possible to demonstrate the production of aggressive behaviour by ESB. It has since become apparent that the aggressive behaviour thus produced may be of two types. In the first instance the animal goes through the motions, as it were, of being aggressive without any evidence of emotional disturbance: such a reaction has been termed "sham rage". In the second instance there is evidence of an emotional response whose behavioural expression may be moderated substantially by the prevailing circumstances.

Thus in discussing such a distinction Delgado (1969) illustrates a form of aggressive expression produced by ESB in the cat. Here the behaviours of hissing, growling etc. appear to represent a "sham rage", not being directed against another cat present at the same time. (Indeed when the other cat responds to this display, the stimulated · cat, far from showing aggression, shows a submissive, defensive posture.) With different stimulation a "true" rage is produced. Here the cat's aggresssive behaviour is clearly directed towards another animal, or towards a human experimenter towards whom the cat was normally friendly. Sham rage, Delgado reports, can be elicited by stimulation of the anterior hypothalamus: "true rage" by stimulation of the lateral hypothalamus.

The effect of the immediate environment on the expression of "true rage" has been described particularly clearly. In one of Delgado's experiments he reports that a monkey given stimulation of the nucleus posterolateralis of the thalamus showed a considerable number of attacks in a social group in which she was normally of high rank, but only one attack in a group where she held low rank.

Numerous studies have shown that aggression can be modified in a number of species by stimulation and/or lesioning of various sites. Particularly common subjects of study are monkeys and cats (both domestic and wild), with the amygdala, thalamus and hypothalamus common sites of stimulation and lesion. Detailed experimentation however has made it abundantly clear that the expression of aggression may depend critically upon specific features of the experimental situation. Thus Delgado (1967) demonstrated that identical stimulation could readily produce aggression between normally friendly cats yet produce no such aggression between normally friendly rhesus monkeys: of possible significance here are the marked differences in social organisation between the two species. Similarly Delgado (1967b) has shown that the same stimulation in the same animal may produce quite different results depending on whether the animal was left free to interact with others, isolated or restrained. Clearly the effect of ESB depends on a constellation of factors.

Inevitably in humans the available evidence is much more sparse. In a study reported by King (1961) a depressed, unemotional psychiatric patient, on stimulation of the amygdala, became highly emotional with signs of increasing anger. On being given a supply of paper she proceeded to tear it to shreds without any prompting. A drop in current intensity from 5 to 4 milliamps resulted in her smiling and attempting to explain herself: return to 5 milliamps resulted once again in the return of the aggresssive behaviour. It is important to note however that, as with the monkey studies, she did not actually attack the experimenter: apparently the normal social constraints on such behaviour were adequate to provide control.

A detailed review of studies linking neurological mechanisms to aggressive behaviour has been presented by Moyer (1971): more recent studies have been summarised by Ursin (1981). Both of these reviews make it clear that the area is highly complex. Ursin (1981) suggests that at least three different types of aggression may need to be distinguished in order to understand the variation in findings from neuroanatomical studies. From the point of view of our present understanding of aggression it would appear that such studies provide clues as to the neural mediation of aggressive behaviour. Perhaps the greatest immediate value of such studies lies in their incidental conclusions: that an understanding of the biology of aggression must still rely upon an understanding of the social and environmental factors involved. As Delgado (1969) has put it "Electricity cannot determine the target for hostility or direct the sequences of aggressive behaviour, which are both related to the past history of the stimulated subject and to ... immediate adaptation to changed circumstances" (page 132).

Just as stimulation of parts of the brain can provide indications of their function, so lesions of the brain have been used to study the role of various structures. As with the stimulation work, and for equally obvious reasons, most of these studies have been conducted with experimental animals, often making generalisation to human aggression difficult.

Much of the work, as may be expected, provides results complementary to the ESB work. Thus in the latter Koolhaas (1978) found that stimulation of the lateral hypothalamus in cats increased some forms of aggression; correspondingly lesions in this area have been found to reduce such behaviour (Adams 1971). Lesions in the posterior hypothalamus, by contrast, have been reported as producing increased aggression (Olivier 1977).

As with the stimulation work, it is not possible here to do more than give a sample of the extensive work that has been conducted in this area: for a more complete review Ursin (1981) should be consulted. Both ESB and lesion studies have implicated a wide range of structures affecting a number of different types of aggressive behaviour. Integration of such studies is often difficult because of the variety of species-specific forms of aggression studied (e.g. frog-killing by rats) and because of the difficulty of distinguishing between changes in aggressiveness as a direct result of lesions and changes which are merely a side effect of other results. As an example of the latter, lesions in the lateral hypothalamus, linked with aggression, are known also to affect systems involved in motivation and perception. It is possible therefore that the changes in aggressive behaviour reflect nothing more than consequences of perceptual and motivational disturbance.

Despite the difficulties of interpreting such carefully controlled laboratory work, a number of workers have made substantial claims for the role of neurological factors. Disturbingly many of these claims seem to be made on the basis of ill-controlled clinical observation, where the number of confounding factors make interpretation even more difficult than in the laboratory. Even more disturbing is the observation that such claims have at times led to the use of neurological approaches to the control of behaviour before the processes involved could reasonably claim too be understood (see Chapter Seven).

Much of the clinical literature seems to be based on the relatively unsystematic observation of associations between disturbed brain funtion and aggressive behaviour. An early example of this is provided by the famous case of Phineas Gage. Phineas was a worker involved in blasting operations in the U.S.A. during the last century. Typically such operations involved the drilling of a hole in rock that was to be blasted. Gunpowder would be inserted into the hole, then a layer of sand, and a metal rod (a "tamping iron") inserted into the hole on top of the gunpowder in order to compress the layer of sand and prevent the blast losing most of its energy back through the hole which had been drilled. Phineas' job was to insert the tamping iron into the hole after the gunpowder and sand had been inserted. Unfortunately on the last of the occasions he did so, the sand had not been poured in. The tamping iron slid into the hole, hit the gunpowder, and was shot straight out again by the resulting explosion. The iron, some 2m long and 2.5 cm in diameter shot through Phineas' head, entering at around the level of the cheekbone, and passing straight through the top of his skull. Perhaps surprisingly Phineas not only survived this injury but was even able to go, with assistance, to the hospital, taking his tamping iron with him. Following treatment he gave up his job (perhaps unsurprisingly) and toured city sideshows, exhibiting his injury and his tamping iron to the public.

The case of Phineas Gage is often quoted as an example of the relationship between brain structure and personality. Although before the accident he was described as pleasant, likeable and easy going, after the accident he was said to become moody, irritable and short-tempered – in short, considerably more aggressive.

It may, however, be a considerable mistake to assume that his personality changes were necessarily a direct result of his brain damage. Leaving aside the possibility that he felt disinclined to trust other people, having been severely injured by another person's carelessness, a number of other factors need to be considered. His injury would, for example, cause considerable disfigurement: could this, rather than the damage to his brain, have been responsible for his change? His leaving his job and joining the sideshows would have produced a substantial change in his lifestyle, social contacts etc. Could this be the cause? It is of course tempting to argue that the neurological trauma must have had some effect on his personality, yet it is generally agreed that it had no effect on his intellectual functioning which, intuitively, one might also have expected to be disrupted. Obviously the changes could be the result of the brain damage, but other explanations are possible.

Such an example shows fairly clearly the dangers of attempting to give definite interpretations to clinical case material. It is now usually accepted that observations on individual clinical cases must be interpreted with caution until more systematic research has been conducted. Such research may substantially alter the initial tentative conclusions. Nevertheless some workers have made substantial claims regarding links between neurological problems and human aggressiveness. Thus Mark and Erwin (1970) noted various parallels between the experiences of temporal lobe epileptics and the experiences commonly preceding violent attacks, suggesting further a frequent coincidence between violent behaviour and temporal lobe seizures. After describing a single case history they concluded that temporal lobe epilepsy was an important example of a known disease state related to violent behaviour.

Systematic research however appears not to support their view. Thus Gunn and Fentin (1971), in a study of 434 temporal lobe epileptics, found violence to be rare. Moreover of 150 cases of epileptics in prison, only 10 reported a seizure within 12 hours of the offence. Brazier (1967) reported that temporal lobe epileptics who had artificial stimulation of various temporal lobe structures never produced a reaction which could be interpreted as anger or fear.

Other brain disorders have also been suggested as possible causes of aggressive behaviour, including rabies, limbic brain tumours and alcohol poisoning. The relevance of these problems to most episodes of violence is however far from clear. Thus not only do most violent individuals show no clear brain pathology, even amongst those with such pathology violence is far from a universal phenomenon. In attempting to justify the inclusion of alcohol in support of an organic model of aggression, some worker have argued for the inclusion of deaths caused by drunken driving in the toll of "violence caused by alcohol": many workers of course feel that such deaths are more a function of loss of skill and reduced concern for safety factors than of any increase in aggressiveness.

This is not to say, of course, that physical problems may not produce aggression and violence as symptoms of the pathology. Physical illnesses with aggression as a symptom, however, seem likely to account for only a small percentage even of the violence found in hospitals: in considering the wider context of violence their role is inevitably relatively small. Moreover the issues involved may be quite straightforward: where physical pathology is identified and treatable this will be desirable irrespective of whether violence forms part of the symptomatology: where there is no evidence of physical pathology it is hard to justify physical intervention. Defenders of psychosurgery now feel unable to support the notion of surgical intervention where there is no underlying brain pathology.

Such viewpoints leave open a third possibility, that of surgical intervention to alleviate aggressive aspects of brain pathology even when the fundamental pathology itself is untreatable. Thus certain types of inoperable brain tumour may bring about behaviour disturbance as a result of increased intracranial pressure. Surgical intervention to relieve such pressure, whilst not curing the underlying pathology, may do much to help the resulting behaviour problems. Such attempts will be considered in more detail later (see Chapter Seven).

THE ETHOLOGICAL APPROACH

One of the most influential approaches to the study of behaviour has been that which has emphasised the observation of behaviour as it occurs in the "natural environment". Inevitably, the behaviour of animals in the wild has been the main focus for this approach and construction upon this methodology has resulted in what we now know as Ethology, greatly popularised by the writings of Desmond Morris and Robert Ardrey. Despite the quite specific misgivings of one of the most influential of ethologists, Tinbergen, that there should be few if any generalisations across species, much has been made of the observations of animals and the interpretations of these for human behaviour, particularly, as it happens, with regard to violent and aggressive behavior. Marsh and Campbell have taken the view that this approach has largely been as a result of the fact that it is well-nigh impossible to simulate aggression and violence in laboratory situations. This, however, serves to justify the methodology of the ethologists rather than the basic tenets of the discipline that much of behaviour comes as specific responses by animals to specific environmental stimuli and that the capacity to respond to these specific stimuli is genetically determined.

It is not surprising then that violent and aggressive behaviour in man, the evidence for which, as we have seen, goes back to the furthest antiquity, should be singled out for particular attention as a prime example of human instinctual behaviour. The idea that human beings behave in a fundamentally instinctual way is a particular ideological concept and it has been argued that the approach of the theory of instinct to human behaviour is a gross over-stretching of the original concepts as applied to animal behaviour. Bernard (1961) listed over six thousand behaviours, specific actions, impulses or motives described variously in the literature as 'instincts'. The point is made that the original concept of 'instincts' being definite, encapsulated and structural has become, in many cases, a whole cluster of behaviours which may become loosely associated according to some form of functional relationship. One of these would become the "instinct of self-preservation"; another would be the "instinct of aggression" and so on

It is possible to identify four main categories of theorist when it comes to the conceptualisation of human behaviour. Whilst this categorisation may be arbitrary, it does describe the range of possibilities. Firstly, there are those theorists who see all behaviour as learned and see "instincts" as being epistemologically irrelevant. The second category would describe those theorists who hold that instincts are important in the lower animals but in human beings we see only the remnants of instincts. Thirdly, we have those who hold that in people there are just a few basic instincts that hold the key to all behaviours and fourthly those who believe that all behaviour is a combination of small instinctual structures. The last three would for some describe the "ethological approach" and the first three for some would describe the "learning approach". Clearly there is a great deal of overlap and we should resist the temptation to over-ideologise. The learning theorist B.F. Skinner, for example, is often quoted as being of the first category yet in his "Contingencies of Reinforcement" (1969) makes the specific point of quoting and supporting Breland and Breland ("No reputable student of animal behaviour has ever taken the position that the animal comes to the laboratory as a virtual 'tabula rasa', that species differences are insignificant and that all responses are about equally conditionable to all stimuli").

What then of the "instinct of aggression" and its consequential violence? Heller, in many ways justifiably, asserts:

> The instinct of aggression...is a bottomless bag into which it is possible to stuff the most diverse behaviours,

attitudes, impulses, activity types,
feelings or character traits. Should
someone commit parricide, slam the
ink-bottle to the floor, play chess, work,
be jealous or envious, take revenge, be
angry, play football or watch the game,
write a book, or...entertain prejudices
...argue...condemn or accuse...prohibit or
act in disregard of prohibition...
revolt...do business, make friends or
love, or...not make friends or not make
love - all of this could be described as a
subtle or not so subtle manifestation
of..(an)...instinct (or drive or motive)
of aggression.

However in this respect the evidence for an instinct
of aggression is no different than the evidence for
an instinct of "maternal care" or an instinct of
"survival".

Nevertheless, humans behave aggressively in
ways which may be seen as similar to the ways in
which animals of other species behave. The approach
of Ethology is to look at the particular behaviours
in particular species and ask general questions
about the functions of these behaviours in terms of
the survival of the species. It may also ask
questions about how the behaviour becomes adapted to
the environment. Obviously, the learning theorist
is also concerned with behavioural adaptation but
the Ethologist would emphasise the genetic
inheritance of behavioural patterns through natural
selection.

Recent observations of groups of
chimpanzees, the species perhaps most closely
related to humans, have produced interesting
speculations regarding adaptive aggressive
behaviour. On the whole, chimpanzees interact with
each other in fairly predictable ways and much of
this interactive behaviour appears to be learned
during growth and development. These social
behaviours are displayed when conditions require
threat, attack, or submission and are most likely
to occur in specific circumstances such as in daily
interactions involving status or dominance, in the
protection of infants by both sexes, in defence
against predators, in terminating disputes or in
circumstances where highly valued resources are in
short supply. We may well see human aggressive
behaviour serving similar functions to the societal
organizations in which we live. It is also of note
that the species which is nearest to us in the

phylogenetic tree:
1) requires particular learning conditions to apply before the behaviour is evident and
2) that the behaviour is considered to be adaptive even when it may involve extreme violence.

However even in chimpanzees we see behavioural patterns which are construed as having the function of inhibiting intra-species aggression. For Lorenz, arguably the most eminent of the ethologists, it is precisely the outstripping of innate inhibitions by rapid technological development of weaponry which makes human beings seem to have such a singular propensity for "intra-specific aggression". Humanity, of course, is not unique in this portrayal of extreme intra-specific aggression. Some tropical fish will eat each other. Lions have been known to kill each other and even the relatively "friendly" chimpanzee will show occasional extreme violence to its fellow in particular circumstances. Nevertheless, it is undeniable that humans are now capable of exhibiting such extreme violence that not only would "homo sapiens" cease to exist but most of the other species of the earth. No one, presumably, would argue that this was "adaptive". Lorenz takes the view that the human being's capacity for conceptual thought and speech has allowed the natural, innate inhibitions shown in the lower animals, to be swamped by the rapid adoption of technological weaponry. When a weapon is invented or discovered, it is possible for this to be immediately incorporated by the entire community, rather than by the mere progeny of the inventor or discoverer. Moreover, the increasing remoteness of the aggressor from the victim prevents any possibility of inhibitory stimuli from taking effect.
The logical conclusion of this is that human beings are doomed to be aggressive and violent because the natural inhibitors are not available as they would have been had the technology of weaponry developed at the pace of natural inheritance. Therefore any attempt to control it should be by diverting this aggressiveness into relatively harmless areas, such as sporting activities. However, this is an extreme view, and not one which is necessarily consistent with the evidence. We cannot claim that all aggressive behaviour is phylogenetically determined. Some may be; this is undeniable. It may be possible for any given instance of aggression to be traced to both kinds of

origin but is important to look for the effective variables which strengthen or weaken aggressive behaviour. The bowing of the head in inhibition of attack, or the baring of the teeth indicating threat may or may not have phylogenetic origins but what is important is that as variables which may functionally relate to aggression, they may have significance in a wider analysis.

PRACTICAL IMPLICATIONS

Despite initial promise as regards the prospect of dealing with problems of aggression it still sems to be the case that biological work is in a fairly early stage of development. Nevertheless it is possible to note at least a few implications of such work for the practical understanding of problems of violence, including:

1. Hormonal investigations have so far failed to establish convincingly a role for such chemicals in the understanding of aggression. To date, the evidence is at least as convincing that aggression causes hormonal variation as vice versa.

2. Similarly the most plausible of theories implicating genetic factors in aggression show only weak or spurious relationships; even where certain genetic problems (e.g. Down's syndrome) seem to be associated with reduced levels of aggression it is still possible to find aggressive individuals with such problems. Conversely where a genetic problem might plausibly seem to be associated with increased aggression (as in the XYY syndrome) it is necessary to avoid being misled by methodological artefacts.

3. Whilst neurological work does much to identify brain structures implicated in aggression, it transpires that even direct manipulation of these structures by ESB or lesion still fails to overcome normal social constraints on violence. The implication is therefore that practical attempts to deal with violence will be much more powerful if based on the environmental context rather than the neurological substrate of the aggression.

4. Direct observation of clinical problems and possible links with aggression may be misleading; whilst the clinic may seem to show an association between such problems as temporal lobe epilepsy and violence, it is difficult to find solid evidence to reinforce such a notion. Clinical material is subject to a number of possible distortions, and notions based purely on clinical impressions without further investigation should be regarded with caution.

5. At a behavioural level biology, through ethology, has generated a good deal of data regarding the occurrence of violence in the natural

environment. Such observations are often construed in terms of an instinctual basis; the concept of instinct is however problematic and it may be appropriate to guard against too hasty an acceptance of such a form of explanation.

Chapter Four

THE SOCIAL/ANTHROPOLOGICAL PERSPECTIVE

In marked contrast to biological accounts of aggression are those based on an anthropological or socio-cultural framework. Where the former have tended to see aggression as, to a large extent, an inevitable part of the human condition, the latter have considered the extent to which violence is a function not of being human, but of living in human society.

Since human biology is largely the same the world over, a purely biological account would imply that violence should itself be similar throughout the world. Since, as we know, societies vary considerably in the extent to which they exhibit violence, it follows that an understanding of violence must extend beyond the purely biological. Much research has therefore been concerned with the cultural variation in violence, with two areas receiving particular study. The first of these concerns what have come to be called 'simple societies', usually involving relatively small numbers of individuals often quite isolated from society at large. A second emphasis has concerned specific subcultures within a larger and more complex society. It is useful to consider these separately.

SIMPLE SOCIETIES

Many anthropologists concerned with the study of simple societies have commented on the role of aggression and violence within these societies. Thus the people of Tahiti have for over 200 years been described by European writers as gentle and peaceful (Levy 1973). Interestingly this "gentle and peaceful nature" appeared not to be part of the

Tahitian biology, but clearly a reflection of culture. In particular the early 19th Century saw reports of violence amongst the Tahitians following cultural changes resulting from Western contact, particularly the impact of Protestant missionaries. That is to say the same people who are gentle and peaceful in one culture can become warlike when the culture changes. A similar change from the peaceful to the warlike was described amongst the Fore of New Guinea with a change from a hunter-gatherer to a settled agriculture form of food production.

Other studies appear to show little or no violence throughout, at least, the periods for which they are studied. Thus in his account of the "stone age" Tasaday, Nance (1975) found no evidence of aggression and indeed entitled his book "The Gentle Tasaday". A study of the Hopi Indians of North America reported that not only did they disapprove of violent acts: even to have violent thoughts could be considered shameful (Brandt 1954). It appears, then, that in some societies at least, aggression and violence are, if not non-existent, at least extremely rare.

At the opposite extreme, some societies have become noted for their extremely warlike and aggressive tendencies. Thus in a study of the Yanomamo Indians of Northern Brazil, Chagnon (1977) noted that violent behaviour could be used to express affection. A Yanomamo woman, for example, would not believe that a man really loved her unless he left her scarred or bruised. The aggressiveness of a culture has of course at times been seen as fulfilling particular social functions. The Crow Indians of North America, for example, showed considerable antagonism towards their neighbours, and in doing so maintained an extremely high level of cooperation and friendliness between themselves. When their warfare was banned by the U.S. Government, one consequence was that they began to quarrel amongst themselves.

This latter observation could of course be used to bolster a notion of "natural aggressiveness". If the Crow were indeed showing a natural biological aggression it would be expected that blocking one outlet for the aggression would lead them to seek another outlet - in this case internal quarrelling. Of course it could simply be that the change merely reflected cultural change involved in the banning of warfare. Certainly it is not the case, as one would expect from a biological explanation, that all attempts to block warfare have resulted in the

finding of "other outlets". Thus the Dani of New
Guinea showed no signs of compensating when warfare
was forbidden. Contrary to the expectations of
anthropologist Karl Heider, the two years following
the banning of warfare showed no abnormal
within-group violence, suicides or sudden increases
in ritual (Heider 1970). Clearly not all violent
societies continue to be violent once the original
form is blocked. Indeed the blocking of fighting in
the Fore culture was welcomed by its members, with a
rapid shift towards an anti-fighting ethic in the
values of the tribespeople.

To some extent these apparently conflicting
findings may not be as paradoxical as they appear.
Thus Blacking (1983) points out that the violence of
the Dani was not a long-standing historical
component of their culture but rather that the Dani
way of life was predominantly peaceful and
non-aggressive, their warlike behaviour representing
a temporarily deviant phase of their history.

The varying degress of aggressiveness do not
appear to relate in any simple way to obvious
variables. Thus differences in the physical
environment do not, alone, appear to explain the
differences in degrees of violence. The violent
Navaho, for example, were near neighbours of the
Hopi, who as we have seen were characteristically
peace-loving. Attempts have been made to explain
the violent behaviour of various groups as adaptive
in terms of their individual circumstances. Harris
(1974) has proposed an explanation of warfare
amongst the Maring of New Guinea in terms of its
overall benefit in ecological and economic terms.
However as Blacking (1983) has pointed out, an
explanation of violence in terms of adaptiveness
still leaves open a number of questions. How, for
example, do people know how much violence or warfare
is adaptive, and when to stop? It is important here
to note that the factors which lead to the
development of warfare may not be the same as those
which subsequently maintain it. Thus warfare may
develop as an adaptation to a particular set of
circumstances, but once established continue for
reasons other than the original ones. In an extreme
case this could lead to warfare becoming established
as an adaptation, changed circumstances later making
it maladaptive but the change away from warfare
occurring too late to avert tragedy. Thus, the
violence of the Yanomamo, whilst posibly adaptive at
one time, is now threatening them with extinction.

What, then, can we learn from the study of

simple societies? One clear lesson is that aggression and violence are not simply part of 'human nature', unless we are to believe that the differing degrees of violence we see reflect different kinds of human beings rather than different cultures. Since we have examples of marked changes in the behaviour of the same human beings when cultural change occurs (as with the Tahitians) we are forced to the conclusion that cultural factors can be a major determinant of aggression and violence.

It is important to note, of course, that cultural factors do not provide a complete account of violence. Thus within a certain culture, some individuals may act in a way quite different to most of the culture's members. Whilst this may to some extent reflect subcultures within the larger culture, even within such subcultures there is considerable variation in the violence of their members (q.v.). Moreover it is also important to remember that much anthropological discussion concerns forms of violence ranging from warfare to individual fighting. To what extent these are simply different extremes of violence, and to what extent they are different kinds may be the subject of disagreement amongst researchers.

On the other hand the fact that cultural factors are clearly capable of playing a substantial role implies that not only must they be taken into account in explaining violence, they must also be considered when evaluating research. Thus although Bolton (1973) claimed a link between blood sugar levels and aggressiveness in the Qolla of Peru, it is important to remember that such a relationship may only be apparent when the cultural conditions are right. Indeed Bolton suspected that the two were connected in a complex interaction rather than in a simple cause – effect manner: that is to say the total stress load (in part, at least, a product of the culture) was seen as the start of a vicious circle of hypoglycaemia and aggressiveness. Clearly in a different culture this cycle may never have become established: in such a culture any variation in blood sugar level may be quite independent of aggressiveness. It should be noted moreover that the existence of any relationship at all between the Qolla's aggression and blood sugar is open to doubt; in a recent review of the relevant evidence Llewellyn (1981) concluded that the Qolla were no more aggressive or homicidal than other groups, that they were no more hypoglycaemic and that "there is little evidence that hypoglycaemia causes aggression".

Of course it is possible to argue that work on such simple societies has little if any relevance for the kind of complex society in which most of us live. In such complex societies, of course, many people are, relatively speaking, fairly non-violent, at least for long periods of time between wars. Nevertheless, within such societies, it has often been possible to identify subgroups whose culture differences produce markedly different levels of violence from the larger society of which they are part.

MORE COMPLEX SOCIETIES

Whilst discussions of simple cultures might seem somewhat distant and unreal to many readers, the same approach to study may be applied to societies of greater complexity. In doing so, two particular perspectives have been of importance: the study of violent subcultures in a relatively less violent society, and comparison of complex societies with respect to their degree of violence. It is useful to consider these in turn.

Violent Subcultures in Larger Society

It will be apparent that, in the kind of society in which most of us live, the degree of aggressiveness of its members is not uniform. Indeed to some extent complex societies seem to mirror the world as a whole, having some subgroups in which violence is common and others in which it is rare. Certain groups (e.g. the Society of Friends or Quakers) may be characterised by extremely low levels of violence: others (e.g. street gangs) by a relatively high level of violence.

A number of researchers have considered the role of sub-cultural factors in delinquency in general and aggression in particular. In one such study (Patrick 1967) a young (and younger-looking) probation officer was able to infiltrate a Glasgow street gang under the pretence of being a borstal boy. As a participant in the gang's activities he was able to observe closely the cultural factors influencing such things as the degree of violence used in particular settings. Patrick found that violence and power were closely related in the gang: a person who confronted or threatened the gang or its dignity would become a legitimate target for subsequent violence. He describes, for example, how one gang member attacked a young woman who had previously laughed at him in the street when wearing the short trousers of his borstal uniform. The fights themselves not uncommonly involved considerable injury and bloodshed, with weapons such as bottles and razors ("shivs") widely used. The violence however was, in general, finely adjusted to the particular situation: absolute, uncontrolled violence was frowned upon and a leader of a gang would not usually be its most violent member. Indeed those individuals whose violence was extreme and uncontrolled were themselves incompletely accepted by the group, becoming known as "nutters". Fear of the consequences of violence was lower than might have been expected: to some extent this may reflect such things as the status granted by battle scars and becoming the centre of attention in the gang upon having a tale to tell of the latest fight. Also of importance was media coverage: a violent incident would result in those involved subsequently scouring the newspapers for reports. The more coverage an incident received, the more status was accorded to those involved.

The picture that emerges is one of violence under the fine control of cultural values. The individuals concerned had mostly learned the 'correct' way to behave in different circumstances. Those who learned best integrated well into the gang, those who were not as expert at matching their behaviour to the value system were less well integrated (e.g. the "nutters"). Such evidence is of course quite consistent with the notion that a culture (or in this case a subculture) exerts a fine degree of control over its members' behaviour.

It is important however to remember that the evidence is limited. Thus in Patrick's study it was only possible to gain entry to the gang by virtue of the fortuitous circumstance of his looking so young (gang members were typically of age 14-15). This makes it difficult to repeat the study in order to allow for such factors as the individual peculiarities of the gang Patrick joined, possible different perceptions of other investigators and so on. It is difficult to assess therefore how much of the evidence would be specific to that particular gang, how much Patrick was influenced by his own expectations etc. There have been other, similar studies (see e.g. Yablonsky's 1962 study of New York street gangs) which, encouragingly, provide similar findings. Inevitably however such studies are infrequent and the evidence they provide must be treated with some caution when it comes to making broader generalisations.

A further problem arises in the interpretation of such work. In the study of simple societies it is difficult to justify physical explanations (e.g. brain damage) of the violence since the physical characteristics of the people under study do not differ in any systematic way from those of other communities. When dealing with a subculture of a larger society, however, it is always possible that the subculture is composed of a different type of individual. It may be, for example, that only those with such physical problems seek out and join groups like gangs. Whilst such an argument is plausible, there are a number of pointers which suggest otherwise. To invoke such an explanation might be seen as unnecessarily complicating the issue: since a cultural explanation is obviously adequate to explain differences in violence between different societies, why should we not regard it as adequate for the subcultures also? Moreover the numbers and ages involved in gangs such as Patrick describes would imply a frequency of such problems at an early age which might seem to many resarchers somewhat implausible. Moreover it seems to be the case that the violence is only apparent whilst the individuals are part of the gang: as they grow too old for the gang their violence also declines. It might of course be tempting to consider the hormonal turmoil of adolescence as responsible, but apart from the fact that adolescents do not show similar violence in other cultures, the beginnings of gang violence were seen by Patrick in small children of around 8 years old.

Perhaps the most important of evidence in such matters however arises when "temporary" subcultures occur with a corresponding "temporary" rise in violence: since no corresponding biological change can be causally identified, this lends strong support to a cultural interpretation. Such temporary subcultures may arise in a number of ways: examples include soldiers going into battle, participants in riots and similar occasions where an individual may be surrounded by others for whom violence is highly valued. Whilst it may be politically expedient to describe the participants in such riots as a minority of extremists, much of the evidence in support of such a view is

unconvincing. Thus Ransford (1968) suggested that
the subjective feeling of powerlessness was a factor
which distinguished those who were willing to use
violence from those who were not. In a study of
U.S. negroes following the Watts riots in 1965
Ransford reported a highly significant relationship
between subjective powerlessness and willingness to
use violence. Whilst his data do indeed indicate
that over 80% of those scoring "low" on his measure
of powerlessness would be willing to use violence,
it is notable that almost 60% of the group scoring
"high" were also willing. Similar results are
apparent for the other two variables for which he
claimed significant associations, "Social contact"
and "Racial dissatisfaction". Even when these
results are combined in a composite score of
alienation there remain a number of exceptions to
the prediction. Thus whilst nearly 90% of the
extremely "non-alienated" were unwilling to use
violence, so were over 75% of the "middle
alienation" group. Even of the highly alienated
group, much smaller than the other two groups, 35%
were still unwilling to use violence. Clearly such
characteristics of the individuals involved fail to
give an adequate account of participation. Taking
however the simpler factor of geographical location,
i.e. whether the people actually lived in the Watts
district or not, re-analysis of the data shows that
taking this factor alone the Watts residents were
more than twice as likely as non-Watts residents to
use violence. Moreover the study was completed
after the riots were over: it seems plausible that
many of the rioters present would have been caught
up in the violence at the time but later regretted
it and hence have gone down as "unwilling to use
violence" despite actually have done so. A similar
sentiment was expressed to the first author by a
long-term prisoner who had participated in a major
riot in a maximum security prison: "everyone else
was doing it and I joined in - it seemed like a good
idea at the time". Before and after the riot this
particular individual had been a well-behaved "model
prisoner". His participation in the riot
constituted his only serious breach of prison
discipline during the whole of his sentence.

    Much evidence seems to suggest that quite
normal, kind and compassionate individuals may
become highly aggressive under the influence of an
appropriate subculture. Experiments in which
subjects have been randomly assigned to one
subculture or another have shown that those assigned

to certain subcultures may show dramatic changes in behaviour. Haney et al.(1973) for example set up a simulated prison in which subjects were randomly assigned to play the roles of prisoner or prison officer. Over a six-day period the two groups, identical to begin with, showed marked differences in behaviour. Subsequent ratings by the "prisoners" described over a third of the "officers" as "extremely hostile, arbitrary and cruel in the forms of degradation and humiliation they invented". Whilst precise interpretation of Zimbardo's results is difficult because of a number of methodological problems, the results are consistent with a view tht cultural and subcultural processes play on important part in determining an individual's behaviour.

Such studies, however, begin to blend with the field of psychology, to be considered in detail in the next chapter. Before proceeding to such an approach it is appropriate to consider briefly some of the characteristics of complex societies as a whole.

Violence and Larger Societies
It is a truism to note that, like the variation in violence between simple cultures, there is considerable variation in violence between more complex cultures. It would generally be agreed, for example, that it is more dangerous to walk through Central Park, New York, after dark, than to take a similar walk through Regents Park, London. Rates of assault, manslaughter, murder, rape and other crimes of violence vary considerably across different countries. Even allowing for differences between the countries in legal processes, recording methods etc., it is clear that some countries are more violent than others. Holland, for example, has a rate of serious offences some 75% less than that of the similar neighbouring province of Nord Rhein Westphalen in Germany. It would be a mistake however to assume that such differences result from profound differences in the type of individuals who live in such countries, or from differences in their physical geographies. Historical reflection indicates that countries may at one period be extremely violent and at others less so. The Germany of today is a long way from the Germany of prison camps and mass extermination; Spain no longer has an Inquisition torturing heretics. The rise and fall of violence in complex societies presents a particular challenge for those attempting to

identify   specific   socio-cultural   factors
responsible. Such studies are not impossible
however: Hovland and Sears (1940) for example, have
linked economic indices to the frequency of
lynchings in the American South. Across different
societies, the relationship between the amount of
combative sport and the amount of violence has been
studied by Sipes (1973). Far from providing an
"outlet" for violence, it was found that those
societies with most combative sport were also those
with most violence. It is of course difficult to
establish causality in such a case: the combative
sport may lead to a higher level of real violence,
or the violence may lead to a greater interest in
combative sport. Or some third factor (e.g. a high
status accorded to "masculine" behaviour) may be
responsible for causing both. Thus although it is
possible to establish that a high level of combative
sport does not eliminate violence, it is not
possible to prove the converse, that such sport
causes violence.

In general it seems clear that studies of more
complex societies mirror the studies of simpler
societies, with tremendous variation between
different cultures, between subcultures of a single
society, and between different periods of the same
society. To the extent that cultural differences
are associated with differences in the level of
violence, it is therefore necessary in understanding
violence to take into account its broader social
content: some people are more violent than others
partly if not largely because they live in a more
violence-orientated society.

PRACTICAL IMPLICATIONS

The study of sociological and cultural influences on behaviour inevitably involves considerable difficulty, not least because the researcher is typically an "outsider" in the culture. Since much of the work depends on observation of correlations, causality may be difficult to determine. Nevertheless the perspective does suggest a number of practical implications including:

1. The observation of societies in which violence is minimal or non-existent shows that it is at least possible for human beings to coexist, and that violence and aggression are not inevitable aspects of "human nature". Whether such peaceful coexistence can be widely achieved however is uncertain. In some societies the peaceful character of its members may for example depend on the presence of a number of superstitious beliefs which would not transfer to other societies.

2. The existence of violent subcultures in larger societies may be a cause for concern if it is accepted that such cultures act as "breeding grounds" for violent acts. The anthropological evidence provides some support for the notion that action should be taken to avoid the formation of such subcultures, in particular by eliminating factors associated with such cultures (e.g. poor housing, overcrowding).

3. The considerable differences in levels of violence between different societies suggests that they should be studied closely in order to find the reasons for such differences. Whilst such studies are likely to be correlational, and hence suggestive rather than conclusive, the evidence may still provide useful guidelines regarding the value or otherwise of certain course of action. The observation that high levels of combative sport correlate with general levels of violence, for example, casts considerable doubt on the notion that "other outlets" should be provided for violence.

4. In terms of a more general understanding of violence, the sociological and anthropological work provides strong evidence that a purely biological explanation is inadequate and emphasises the need for careful study of cultural and subcultural factors in violence.

Chapter Five

THE PSYCHOLOGICAL PERSPECTIVE

Biological research being, at best, of limited applicability, and anthropological work indicating the tremendous variability of aggressive behaviour, it seems natural to enquire about the psychological processes involved in aggression. Aggressive behaviour has in fact been studied by a number of psychologists from many different backgrounds including the clinical, observational and experimental. Of particular interest here have been the study of ways in which the individual's interaction with the environment may produce violence; attention has also been directed to the identification of psychological characteristics of violent people. In addition a number of studies have investigated methods of treating violent people using psychological methods (see Chapter Seven). Such interest in the causes and treatment of violence can be traced back at least as far as the work of Freud.

FREUD'S THEORIES OF AGGRESSION

It is interesting that even the great Sigmund Freud found the analysis of violence particularly difficult, despite devoting considerable effort and attention to the problem. His notion of libidinous energy, a striving of the individual towards pleasurable and enjoyable experiences, proved remarkably difficult to reconcile with a number of phenomena and as a result he felt it necessary to postulate a second drive, "Thanatos", being not a seeking after pleasure but a drive towards death and destruction. The organism, Freud postulated, was in a state of permanent tension resulting from its divergence, through life, from its original non-living state. Whilst this energy could be released through the destruc tion of the individual, Freud also felt that it could be redirected and put to different uses in much the same way that Eros, the pleasure principle, could be redirected. One such redirection, Freud argued, would be towards others instead of the self, and outwardly directed aggression would result.

Obviously such a theory has a number of problems, particularly in dealing with anthropological evidence of totally non-violent cultures (see Chapter Four). The observation that high levels of combative sport, far from discharging aggressive drives, are associated with high levels of violence in the culture, casts doubt on the notions of aggressive energy. Freud himself was never totally happy with the theory and subjected it to a number of revisions throughout his life. His views on the possibility of eliminating aggression were basically pessimistic: people were naturally aggressive, and the only way to relieve aggression would be to redirect the aggressive energy. In a famous open letter to Albert Enstein on the subject of war, Freud suggested that much of the hope lay in the possibility of redirecting the aggressive energy to the formation of positive emotional bonds between people. Exactly how this was to be done was never entirely clear, although in the same letter Freud appeared to place much emphasis on the hope for a "cultural evolution" which would produce a society in which the individual's aggression would be brought under the control of a strong superego. Such a notion remains essentially pessimistic, implying that people will not stop wanting to be aggressive, only that such urges can be held in check. The notion of a society in which there would be no urge to aggression seems to be too much to hope for.

In general Freud's theory has failed to gain wide acceptance amongst those concerned with aggression: even some of his closest adherents have suggested that it is of little therapeutic relevance, despite its appeal to fashionable intellectuals: as Stafford-Clarke (1967 p. 159) put it, the theory "proved of far more use to artists and novelists than to clinicans".

Whilst Freud was struggling to produce a satisfactory psychoanalytic theory of aggression, however, psychology was developing a range of instruments and tests to assess such characteristics as intelligence, personality etc. Such an approach led naturally to attempts to produce analyses of aggression in terms of the personality characteristics of violent individuals.

PERSONALITY THEORIES

One of the first substantial attempts to link personality characteristics with aggression came from Eysenck's (1964) work which attempted to link criminality to personality traits which could be measured using pencil and paper tests. In its simplest form Eysenck's theory assumes that the individual learns a "conscience" by which aggression is controlled, through a process of conditioning, such conditioning often being assumed to be Pavlovian in nature. (Such an assumption would of course be regarded as highly suspect by many workers.) Personality characteristics associated with conditionability would therefore be similarly associated with criminality: the extrovert, who is difficult to condition, would be less likely to learn right from wrong and hence more likely to indulge in delinquent behaviour (Eysenck 1983). The theory has been subject to a number of revisions but retains a number of problems, both as a theory of criminality and, of relevance here, as a theory of violence. With regard to the latter it is notable that Eysenck makes little distinction between crime in general and violent crime in particular. The theory has largely been tested on violent offenders, with little attention to the kind of "social violence" described in Chapter Two. Even when applied purely to individuals in custody researchers have often failed to obtain the expected results (Hoghughi and Forrest 1970).

The application of personality assessment to problems of violence in particular has however raised some interesting and promising possibilities. In one of the most well thought out perspectives Megargee (1966) distinguished two possible sources of violent behaviour within the individual from quite different personality types. The first of these types, which Megargee refers to as "undercontrolled", is the type of individual who, as the name implies, makes little or no attempt at self-control when in an aggression-inducing situation. Such an individual will respond aggressively where others would not, purely as a result of minimal self-restraint. As a result such individuals would present with a history of a number of violent episodes and would be characterised by the ease with which violent behaviour could be elicited.

The second type of individual, in whom Megargee expresses particular interest, shows just the opposite pattern of behaviour. Such an "overcontrolled" individual will hold aggression in check in situations where most individuals would react violently. In his original exposition of the theory Megargee discussed this in terms of an accumulation of undischarged violent energy as a period of time, such energy eventually being too much to control and resulting in a violent outburst. Whilst the notions of "aggressive energy" reminiscent of Freud's Thanatos may seem to raise the same kinds of difficulties as a Freudian theory, such a notion is not essential to the general framework and the data can well be accommodated without recourse to such problematic concepts. A number of studies of extremely aggressive offenders have indeed found links between the overcontrolled personality and episodic extreme violence (e.g. Blackburn 1968). Certain individuals, it would appear, are normally non-violent but suddenly and unexpectedly may commit an act of quite extreme violence, often disproportionate to the provocation. That the individual eventually encounters a situation where self-control becomes inadequate is perhaps unsurprising. Most of us do not have to suffer any kind of strong provocation since we tend to suppress such provocation at an early stage. To the extent that we use mild forms of aggression to do so, it is to be expected that we will be more successful than the overcontrolled individual who fails to suppress the first signs of provocation in others in the way that many people would. Overcontrolled individuals, then, will be more likely than the rest of us to be exposed to extended or intense provocation. Eventually such provocation may reach a point where even the overcontrolled's degree of self-control is inadequate and violence results.

An additional factor is introduced by the fact that the overcontrolled individual, unlike others, has little "practice" at being violent. Most people, as a result of such practice, become quite skilled at matching their aggressive responses to the demands of the situation (a violent blow to an attacking mugger but only a mild reprimand to a nagging child). The overcontrolled individual, however, may be likely to "mismatch" the response and the situation, producing a degree of violence quite disproportionate to the eliciting events.

The theory associating over- and under-control with violent behaviour thus has a plausible basis and a degree of empirical support. This is not to say that it is without its problems however. For example, although the studies may tell us that a number of violent people are overcontrolled, the converse question, of how many overcontrolled people are violent, remains unanswered. That is to say we do not know how many overcontrolled people there are in society at large, quietly living their lives without ever indulging in any violence, perhaps never being exposed to situations where violence is called for. The general nature of over- and under-control is far from clear. Does it refer to a broad personality characteristic, or is the individual merely overcontrolled with respect to violence? Whatever kind of characteristic it is, does it remain stable through an individual's lifetime, or may someone change? If the latter, what processes may produce such a change, and if the change occurs does it produce a corresponding change in the probability of extreme violence? Whilst tentative answers can be given to some of these questions, much remains to be clarified.

Implicit in the above discussions has been the notion that an individual's violence is not merely a function of being over- or under-controlled, but also of the particular situation. More precisely, the behaviour depends on both the situation and what the individual brings to that situation: these two are of course likely to interact in possibly complex ways. Much of psychology's research into personality was discouraged when it became clear that even the best information regarding an individual's personality was relatively unhelpful in predicting what an individual would do. By comparison information regarding the situation often provides a much better basis for prediction (see e.g. Mischel 1967). That is to say, in predicting how a person will behave, it is much more useful to know about the situation than the individual's personality. Under certain circumstances the most placid of individuals may become violent, and of course even the most violent of individuals are non-violent for most hours of the day. As a result of considerations such as this attempts have been made to determine the situational factors involved in aggressive behaviour, giving rise to a large body of experimental work.

EXPERIMENTAL STUDIES

In one of the earliest theories attempting to identify situational determinants of aggression, Dollard et al. (1939) postulated a link between frustration and aggression, such that an individual who was frustrated in attempting to achieve some goal would respond aggressively. In a number of experimental studies it was shown that experimentally induced frustration could greatly increase the likelihood of aggressive behaviour. In such studies frustration has usually taken the form of blocking the subject's access to some desired goal, normally when the subject is already some way along the behaviour sequence leading to it. For example a subject may be given a puzzle to solve and then interrupted and moved to another task just before the solution was reached. Children may be shown a playroom containing a number of attractive toys, only to have them removed once access to the playroom is granted. Besides such "response blocking" procedures, researchers have also used punishers (e.g. an insulting experimenter), delay of reinforcement (keeping the individual waiting) and other forms of frustration. All have been shown to increase aggressiveness on a number of measures including direct observation, situational test, self-rating of hostility etc. Such studies led Dollard et al. (1939) to the conclusion that "aggression is always a consequence of frustration". Such a theory turns out however to be a little ambiguous: does it say that whenever aggression occurs it should always be possible to identify some frustrating circumstance which has given rise to it? Or does it· say that whenever frustration occurs it will inevitably result in aggression? The first interpretation holds open the possibility that sometimes frustration will occur without aggression resulting, the second holds out the possibility that whilst frustration will always result in aggression, there may be other processes which might also be implicated instead (or as well). In their original paper Dollard et al. seem to be suggesting a precise one-to-one correspondence between frustration and aggression with one never occurring without the other. Later Miller (1941) seems to imply that frustration always leads to the urge to aggress but that the expression of this urge will depend on a number of other factors as well.

Whichever interpretation is taken the theory has certain problems in its strongest form. Certainly frustration does not always lead to aggression (the urge to aggression is of course something of which we could never directly know the existence). A number of alternative consequences to frustration have also been noted including regression in young children (i.e. exhibiting behaviour which is relatively immature) withdrawal from the situation, and help-seeking behaviour (Bandura 1973). As we shall see later it also seems to be the case that aggressive behaviour can be produced without any prior frustration, e.g. by learning to aggress in order to obtain some reward. Because of this latter possibility Dollard et al. found it necessary to exclude specifically such "instrumental aggression" from their theory. Nevertheless a considerable amount of research has shown some links between frustration of goal-seeking behaviour and aggressive behaviour, and it would of course be foolhardy to neglect such research. It seems clear however that the picture is much more complex than Dollard et al. suggested, and that other factors may also have to be taken into consideration.

Of particular relevance to the study of frustration and aggression has been subsequent experimental work on the eliciting of aggressive behaviour by various kinds of stimulus. From such a viewpoint frustration may be seen as just one of the events which may produce and aggressive reaction. The use of a more general category of "reactive aggression" to cover occasions where the aggression is elicited by some prior event may make the separate consideration of frustration unneccesary.

REACTIVE AGGRESSION

A considerable amount of research suggests an extension to the frustration-aggression hypothesis to the effect that aggressive behaviour may occur as a reaction to aversive events of many kinds, frustration being only one example. Because of the nature of this relationship such aggression has been termed "reactive aggression" (Owens and Bagshaw 1984), being a reaction to some prior stimulation.

In a classic study Ulrich and Azrin (1962) showed that it was possible to produce fighting in experimental animals in response to an aversive stimulus like an electric shock. In the basic experiment two rats were placed in an experimental chamber from which they could not escape. Normally the rats showed no signs of hostility towards each other; however when an electric current was applied to the cage floor the rats adopted a stereotyped fighting posture, rising on their hind legs and striking each other with their forepaws. The response seems to be a fundamental and strong aspect of the animal's make-up. Ulrich and Azrin were able to demonstrate the effect repeatedly at high shock frequencies until the animals literally became too exhausted to fight. The effect of changing a number of the experimental parameters was closely investigated. Changing the strain or sex of the animal used had no effect on the reliability of the response; neither did giving the animals time in each other's company prior to the experiment (to increase their familiarity). Changing the aversive stimulus did however have an effect, particularly in that reducing the strength of the shock reduced the reliability with which the response could be obtained. From this a general conclusion seemed to be that aggressive behaviour could occur as a reaction to prior aversive stimulation; the more severe the stimulation, the more likely the aggression.

Because of the characteristics of the original studies such a response was labelled "shock-induced fighting" or "shock-induced aggression". Subsequent experiments have however shown that the same response can be elicited by many kinds of aversive stimulus besides electric shock. The fact that frustrating situations could elicit aggressive reactions was of course already known; in addition other aversive stimuli may also do so. In particular it should be noted that the response can be elicited by stimuli whose aversive properties have been learned by the subject as well as stimuli which are intrinsically aversive. Thus if a neutral stimulus (e.g. a tone or a light) precedes shock, this stimulus will eventually come to elicit fighting in a manner similar to the shock itself (Vernon and Ulrich 1966). Since the same process seems to be capable of initiation by a number of kinds of stimulus besides shock, the term "shock-induced" may be unneccessarily specific and potentially misleading. Such a term as "reactive aggression" is therefore preferable, being more general and reflecting what appears to be a commonality of process in the various experiments.

Since the original study was conducted the same process has been demonstrated with a wide range of species including birds, fish, primates etc. The general finding to emerge is that over a wide range of species aggressive behaviour can be elicited by stimuli which are aversive to the individual concerned. The process is sensitive to certain parameters, including changes in shock intensity as described above. Where escape from the aversive stimulus is possible, this appears prepotent over fighting. Certain drugs appear to affect the probability of fighting in response to aversive stimulation. In general however the phenomenon seems to be a strong component of the behaviour of most species and offers a possible framework for the consideration of much human aggression. Parallels can be seen in anecdotal, clinical and experimental studies of human aggression. At a simple level Seligman (1975) has pointed out that the phenomenon is familiar to anyone whose head is hit by the car door on entering, and who subsequently becomes furious, yelling at the passengers. Clinically the occurrence of aggressive behaviour has been observed following the withdrawal of the normally rewarding consequences of a behaviour (see e.g. Chapter Nine), a process which has also been demonstrated experimentally (e.g. Kelly and Hake 1970). The process of reactive aggression, then, provides the beginning of a framework within which to consider psychological aspects of violence.

As with the original frustration-aggression theory, however, it is clear that such a process is inadequate as an explanation of all aggressive behaviour. Much aggression seems to reflect the way in which certain individuals have learned to achieve their desired goals rather than an inbuilt response to some unpleasant antecedent. For this reason it is important to consider aggression as a learned behaviour, as well as aggression as a natural part of the organism's functioning.

LEARNING PROCESSES IN AGGRESSION

We have already seen that learning may play a part in reactive aggression, in that such aggression may be elicited by a stimulus whose aversive properties have been induced by a conditioning process. Learning however seems to be relevant in not only the production of links between neutral and aversive stimuli but also in the production of aggressive behaviour itself.

Much aggressive behaviour, indeed, appears not

to be elicited by any particular prior stimulus but rather to represent an attempt to obtain some subsequent goal. That is to say, the behaviour appears to be more under the control of consequences than antecedents.

Where behaviour is primarily under the control of its usual consequences it is usually considered to be an example of operant conditioning. This type of conditioning, to be distinguished from Pavlovian conditioning, is concerned with the ways in whch individuals learn to behave in particular ways in order to achieve certain results. An important class of such consequences is that known as reinforcers, or strengtheners of the behaviour. Thus a hungry pigeon which receives food when it pecks at a disc on the wall of its cage is more likely to do it again than one which does not receive food. Most studies of operant behaviour have been concerned with such responses as the pecking of discs by pigeons or the pressing of levers by rats, since such behaviours are easy to measure and study. A number of studies have however demonstrated similar processes in human subjects, suggesting that the results may perhaps be extended across species.

Although operant conditioning studies typically involve some arbitrarily selected behaviour, usually chosen for ease of recording, the same process has been shown to be capable of producing specifically aggressive behaviour. Establishment of behaviours of varying degrees of complexity has been possible with operant conditioning. In one procedure reinforcers are initially delivered for any behaviour which even vaguely resembles the desired, final behaviour. As such vaguely similar behaviour becomes more common the criteria for reinforcement become more stringent, only those instances where the behaviour is reasonably similar to the eventual target being reinforced. In this way much of the subject's behaviour becomes close to that desired; momentary variations in the behaviour make it possible to reinforce differentially closer and closer approximations to the final behaviour until the required form is achieved. Such a procedure, known as "shaping" (from the way the behaviour is gradually "shaped" to the final form) has been widely used both in the training of experimental animals (e.g. Skinner 1938) and in the teaching of new skills in clinical settings (e.g. Mikulas 1972).

By using such a shaping procedure it has been possible to produce in experimental subjects aggressive behaviour which is under reinforcement control. Thus Reynolds, Catania and Skinner (1963) and Azrin and Hutchinson (1967) were able to produce an increased likelihood of aggressive behaviour in pigeons using food as a reinforcer. In human subjects too, reinforcement seems to be capable of affecting the likelihood of aggressive behaviour. Thus Walters and Brown (1963) showed that reinforcement of the aggressive behaviour of a group of boys led to a subsequently higher level of aggression than was observed in a similar group where aggression was not reinforced. In the natural environment, of course, aggressive behaviour often leads to reinforcement. Thus Patterson et al. (1967) showed that counter-attack by victimised children in nursery school increased in frequency if they were successful. That is to say reinforcement of the counter-attack (by driving away the attacker) led to an increased frequency of its occurrence.

A number of workers (e.g. Owens and Bagshaw 1984) have pointed out that reinforcers maintaining aggressive behaviour may be relatively arbitrary or may have an obvious and intrinsic relationship to the behaviour. Thus attacking a victim may produce a number of consequences such as crying, defensiveness, submission etc. which may serve reinforcing functions for some individuals and hence help to maintain such behaviour in the attacker. Such consequences are in a sense intrinsic to the type of behaviour in question (i.e. aggressive behaviour) and bear an obvious relationship to it. On the other hand aggressive behaviour may also be reinforced by arbitrary consequences which, whilst desirable from the attacker's point of view, bear no logical relationship to the type of behaviour. Thus the food with which Azrin and Hutchinson (1967) reinforced attack behaviour in pigeons would not constitute a form of reinforcement intrinsic to aggressive behaviour in the same way that signs of hurt on the victim would. The implication is that aggressive behaviour may be maintained by both natural and arbitrary reinforcement. In the natural environment arbitrary reinforcers such as food and sexual contact may be of particular importance where there is competition for limited resources. Other arbitrary reinforcers may also be implicated however, including status, prestige and (in such cases as organised crime) money: the role of such factors has been discussed in detail by Buss (1971).

STIMULUS VARIABLES IN OPERANT BEHAVIOUR

It is important to note, however, that operant behaviour may occur not only as a direct result of the effects of reinforcers but also as a result of changes in stimulus conditions. The most obvious example of this occurs when a new behaviour is learned directly through the imitation of others. That is to say an individual may learn to copy behaviour exhibited by another individual "modelling" such behaviour. In a number of studies on such processes Bandura (1959, 1973) has pointed to the importance of modelling or imitation as a factor in the production of aggressive behaviour. Adolescent boys who were aggressive, for example, were more likely to have parents who used physical punishment than were non-aggressive boys, suggesting that the punishment, far from eliminating the aggression, had actually provided a model for the boys to copy. In a series of experiments Bandura was able to show that children who had observed aggressive behaviour by adults (either in real-life or on film) were more likely to show aggression in a test situation than children who had not seen a model.

Such awareness of the role of imitation has led to a considerable amount of research on the effects of observing violence on subsequent aggressive behaviour. It is clear that imitation itself can be brought under reinforcement control, such that an individual will imitate another as long as such imitation brings success, imitation ceasing after a while if the imitation fails to be reinforced. A number of characteristics of the model seem to affect the probability of imitation occuring. Important amongst these are the extent to which the model is similar to the observer, the extent to which there exist situational similarities between that modelled and that observed, and whether or not the model's behaviour is itself seen to be reinforced (e.g. Bandura Ross and Ross 1963).

Research on imitative behaviour has given rise to considerable concern regarding the effects of such things as television and film violence. Such research is too voluminous for consideration here, but a good review may be found in Brody (1977). In general research on this topic has been inconclusive, the effects being sensitive to a number of important variables. One such variable, the total amount of exposure to the material, may be of particular importance with the development of the

home video industry. In the past film and
television violence, if frequent, has at least been
fairly brief. Since home videotapes permit the
continual playing and replaying of scenes of
violence it is possible that their effects may be
greater. Certainly anecdotal evidence suggests that
films with a predominantly violent content account
for a substantial percentage of the films borrowed
from video libraries.

Disturbingly a second variable relevant to the
availability of video films may be of some
importance. Research on screen violence has often
suggested that the violence seen is not perceived as
'real' by the viewer, with the implication that
unreal violence is less likely to be influential.
The appearance of what have come to be called
"snuff" videos (from the title of one of the first
examples) may be important here. In such films the
violence portrayed is claimed by the producers to be
genuine, filming having occurred "where life is
cheap". The influence of such material has yet to
be subject to detailed study.

Stimulus factors may of course affect operant
behaviour in other ways than providing a basis for
imitation. Much of our behaviour is learned through
such processes as verbal instruction, and very often
our decision to act is one way or another affected
by stimuli which are present. A decision to attack
another individual, for example, may be influenced
by noting the presence of several of the
individual's friends who would be likely to restrain
an attack making it unlikely to succeed.

To the extent that a stimulus (or complex of
stimuli) affects the probability of certain
behaviour occurring, that stimulus is said to exert
control over the behaviour (Terrace 1966). A
considerable body of research has shown that control
over a behaviour will be established by stimuli
which indicate changes in the reinforcement
contingencies. Thus if a behaviour is reinforced in
the presence of a red light but not in the presence
of a green one, the colour of the light will exert
control over the behaviour; the behaviour will be
more likely to occur in the presence of the red
light than the green.

Stimuli which exert control over operant
behaviour are known as discriminative stimuli, since
they provide a means of discriminating between
reinforcement conditions. Such stimuli may affect
the probability of aggressive behaviour in a number
of ways. To have a friend offering support if an

attack takes place is to obtain an indication that
reinforcement is more likely, and hence to increase
the probability of attack. Other stimuli may serve
to indicate that reinforcement is less likely, as in
the example of the presence of the victim's friends.
Under such circumstances the probability of attack
decreases. In any practical situation the
probability of violence occurring will thus be a
complex function of the combined effects of
different discriminative stimuli, some increasing
the probability of violence and some decreasing it.

One set of discriminative stimuli which has been
closely studied for their effects on aggressive
behaviour is that of weapons. Whilst it would be
unsurprising to find that a weapon in the hands of a
potential victim reduced the probability of
aggression (by indicating a reduced probability of
reinforcement) with a converse effect when in the
hands of an aggressor, the role of weapons may be a
little more complex. In a series of experiments
Berkowitz and his co-workers have shown that the
presence of a weapon, even if not actually available
to an individual, can still result in increased
aggressiveness. In one experiment, for example,
Berkowitz and LePage (1967) obtained greater
aggression from angered subjects in the presence of
weapons (a revolver and a shotgun) than when weapons
were absent, even though the weapons were not
actually available to the subject. No such effect
was found for non-angered subjects. The results
appear to imply that weapons alone will not actually
produce aggression, but where aggression is made
more likely (by angering the subject) the presence
of weapons may increase its probability. Such an
effect has been termed the "weapons effect" and
explained in terms of providing an associative cue
prompting aggressive behaviour. The weapons effect
has however proved remarkably difficult to replicate
(e.g.Buss, Booker and Buss 1972) and many
researchers have concluded that the effect is weak
or is merely an experimental artefact (for a fuller
discussion see Zillman 1979 pp. 146-157). In the
present state of knowledge it is difficult to say
for certain that weapons have an effect above and
beyond the effect of any other discriminative
stimuli.

INTERACTIONS OF PSYCHOLOGICAL PROCESSES

Experimental research, then, suggests two quite

independent routes to aggressive behaviour. The first is through the process of operant conditioning: here we might include the violence of the armed robber, or that of the boxer. The behaviour is relatively unemotional and is performed in the hope of gaining some clearly achieveable end: there may be no specific prior stimulus discernible to which the aggression can be said to be a response. The second type of aggression, by contrast, is in clear response to some prior unpleasant event: here we might include the aggression of the individual whose toe is accidentally trodden on, or the person who reacts violently to hearing of the death of a loved one.

In many cases of aggression both processes will combine and interact. Thus the ethologists (see Chapter Three) have described at some length the phenomenon of "territorial aggression". This refers to the aggression directed by some species towards intruders into an area set aside as their territory. Here it seems likely that the two processes described above are interacting. The intrusion of another creature into the animal's territory may be seen as an aversive event. If this is so, then by the process of reactive aggression we would expect an aggressive response (to give up one's territory is almost certain to be even more aversive, so escape is not a possibility). The general effect of such aggression is to drive away the intruder: the aggression is thus reinforced and more likely to recur in the future. A similar combination of processes is apparent in much human aggression. One person may annoy another and thereby produce reactive aggression. If this leads to the annoyer being driven away, or otherwise to the cessation of the annoyance, the reactive aggression will be reinforced, producing a combination of reactive and operant processes.

Such interactions may be particularly complex when considering more than one individual. Street and pub fights, for example, typically develop through a rapid escalation of threats, gestures and violent acts. The slight threat made by one individual may elicit aggressive behaviour from the other. Such behaviour may itself elicit further aggression from the first leading to a cycle of escalation within a reactive process. Recognition that the other person has indeed been annoyed may also in many cases provide reinforcement, again leading to a cycle of rapid escalation. In such circumstances the presence of an audience may also

provide further reinforcement and discriminative
stimuli with consequent further acceleration of the
escalation. Such influences from extraneous factors
(like a social group) highlight the fact that the
basic processes, once set in motion, may be subject
to influence from a number of extraneous variables.

FACTORS WHICH MODERATE BASIC PROCESSES

Whilst it appears that for violence to occur either
a reactive or operant process must be involved, it
is clear that a number of factors, not sufficient to
produce violence by themselves, are nevertheless
capable of influencing the basic process. Obvious
influences occur when the factor provides sources of
discriminative stimuli and reinforcement (as with a
social group) but other factors may also be
involved. Such factors may have quite distinct
effects on the two processes.

THE SOCIAL ENVIRONMENT

Much research, both experimental and ethological,
attests to the influence of the social environment
on aggressive behaviour. Such a variable can be
seen to have several opportunities to influence
aggressive behaviour. Thus in a reactive fighting
process the presence of a social group may serve to
intensify the aversiveness of trigger stimuli (e.g.
by implying some kind of public humiliation). Such
a social group will thus increase the probability of
reactive fighting occurring. Conversely some social
groups, for example a peer group consisting of
pacifists, may serve to indicate punishment of
aggression, or to indicate that aggressive behaviour
may not be possible. Under such circumstances there
is evidence to suggest that reactive aggression will
be inhibited.
    Thus with respect to reactive aggression it is
not possible to make an unequivocal statement
regarding the effect of the social environment
without specifying precisely the detailed functions
of that specific social group for the individual
concerned.
    A similar position obtains in the consideration
of operant aggression. Here we can identify several
possible roles of a social environment including a
source of punishment or reinforcement, possibly
intense and immediate, and a source of a number of

discriminative stimuli. These latter may serve to increase or decrease the probability of aggressive behaviour depending upon their relationship to the contingencies operating. Thus a group of fellow football supporters may indicate a potentially high level of reinforcement contingent on aggression: a group of policemen on the other hand may indicate to the same individual a high probability of punishment. Again it is clear that with respect to operant aggression the effects of a social group are complex and will depend on the functional significance of the group for the individual concerned.

As with reactive aggression, it seems likely that reinforced aggression may be affected through a social group moderating the effects of other variables as, for example, when interpersonal dominance serves also to impress an audience or when membership of a large group gives an air of immunity from punishment ("safety in numbers"). A more subtle aspect of this operates when the presence of others indulging in violence serves to influence the individuals' value system, making violence less susceptible to self-control via self-punishment.

Finally, of course, the social group serves as a rich source of verbal guidelines or "rules" of behaviour. It is important to note here that much human aggression is probably controlled by the cultural norms of society which proscribe undue violence. Such "rules of behaviour" are rarely explicit and common to all members of society. Rather each member is likely to generate a personal set of rules reflecting individual experiences within that society. Such rules may exert only a weak control, reflecting the inconsistency of real-life contingencies. It follows that such rules will be particularly susceptible to modification or disruption in a subgroup with immediate and consistent rules which conflict with those of the individual. As a result individuals in certain social groups may modify quite dramatically their views of what is "right" and "wrong", with obvious implications for self-control in aggression.

OTHER FACTORS

Obviously many of the factors already discussed may serve to affect basic processes. Thus certain hormones may be implicated in aggressive behaviour, administration of hormones affecting the likelihood of aggression. Such factors as a history of overcontrolled or undercontrolled behaviour may also modify the extent to which aggression is observed under particular circumstances. In any real situation, therefore, there will exist a number of factors which will interact with basic processes to provide a highly complex picture, some factors intensifying the basic processes, some alleviating them, some having different effects on each basic process and some affecting other external factors. In attempting to understand such a picture, therefore, it is necessary to look not only at what factors may be involved but also at how they may interact.

PRACTICAL IMPLICATIONS

The long history of psychological research has been coupled with a strong practical emphasis. Each of the different perspectives within psychology has implications for the practitioner, including:

1. Whatever the intuitive appeal of a concept like "Thanatos", an instinct to death and destruction, it appears to be of little practical value even to those who are otherwise strongly committed to a Freudian approach. It is of course also difficult to reconcile with much of the anthropological evidence.

2. Research on the "aggressive personality" has had varying degrees of success. Notions of overcontrol and undercontrol emphasise that not all violence is similar in its origins. In particular it is clear that the kind of treatment one might adopt for the overcontrolled individual would be quite different to that of the undercontrolled. As yet, personality research is not sufficiently far advanced to permit prediction of which individuals will or will not become violent.

3. Despite the difficulties of early work based on notions of "frustration" experimental work has had a substantial impact on our understanding of aggression. The identification of distinct processes (reactive and operant) implies that "aggression" should not be treated as a single entity. Evaluation of theorising, research and treatment in the area of aggression should be closely examined in order to determine exactly which process is involved.

4. The role of discriminative stimuli in aggression implies that learning of aggressive behaviour may take place by observation of the aggression of others, a notion supported by a good deal of experimental work. It is to be expected however that such learning will be sensitive to a number of other factors.

5. Besides acting individually the two basic processes may also interact with each other, both being involved in any single episode. In addition a number of other factors may affect the basic processes. The social environment in particular provides a source of various reinforcers,

discriminative stimuli etc. the immediacy of many of these implying the possibility of a powerful influence on behaviour.

Chapter Six

TOWARDS AN INTEGRATION OF DIFFERENT PERSPECTIVES

In the preceding chapters we have seen how workers
with different perspectives and backgrounds have
offered a number of diverse accounts of violent
behaviour. Thus the biologists have referred to
such things as genetics, hormonal factors and so on
to account for aggression. Sociologists and
anthropologists have indicated the extent to which
human beings vary in aggressiveness according to
social and cultural factors. Similarly
psychologists have pointed to such things as
situational determinants, personality factors and
the like in explaining violence.

It is important to remember that, whether or not
the theoretical models of each of these workers is
in agreement, each has provided factual information
which needs to be incorporated in any overall theory
of aggression. It should be possible, therefore, to
provide an analysis of aggression which takes
account of information from each of these sources,
incorporating them into a single coherent model of
aggressive behaviour.

In the present state of our knowledge, of
course, any such overall model must necessarily be
somewhat tentative. Controversy still reigns over
the exact significance of much of the data and the
role of some factors is still far from clear.
Nevertheless there are certain advantages to
producing at least a preliminary integration of
different approaches into a single model. These
include:

i. The more complete the model the better our
ability to understand behaviour. Thus in a purely
psychological model we can explain aggressive
behaviour occurring in response to certain aversive
stimuli (see Chapter Five). If however we extend
the model to incorporate physiological factors we

may note that this reaction becomes more likely when certain drugs are used. By combining the physiological and the psychological we are able to increase our ability to understand the violent behaviour.

ii. In a similar way, by increasing the range of factors included in our understanding of aggression, we are better able to predict violence. Thus noting that an individual is from a social group or culture where violence is common may lead us to predict a higher likelihood of violence than would be expected from another individual who is not from such a culture. By identifying the role of such additional factors as reinforcement schedules we may extend our general prediction (that the person is more likely than another to be violent), to actually predict some of the situations in which that person may actually exhibit violence. Thus combining the anthropological and the psychological we are better able to predict behaviour.

iii. Finally by identifying a wide range of possible variables, greater scope is provided for dealing with the problem. The theorist who sees violence in purely physiological terms is limited to physiological solutions. Similarly sociological analyses indicate only sociological solutions. By extending the number of factors incorporated into the model it becomes possible to select from a wider range of options for dealing with the problem.

It should be noted, incidentally, that what is being suggested here is not a call for "eclecticism". "Eclectics" was the name given to ancient Greek philosophers who, having no system of their own, simply took the parts they liked best of other schools of thought and lumped them together without attempting to integrate them into a system of their own. Many clinicians claim similarly to be "eclectic", taking parts of different schools of thought without any attempt at integration, an approach which has been criticised elsewhere (e.g. Owens 1976). The present approach, by providing an integration of the different approaches, is not eclectic, but rather a synthesis.

Such an attempt obviously cannot be done by clinging to only one of the perspectives outlined earlier. What is needed is a means of integration which will cut across the disciplinary boundaries enabling data from a wide range of sources to be combined within a single model. Such a possibility is provided by the procedure which has come to be known as functional analysis.

FUNCTIONAL ANALYSIS

The term functional analysis refers to an approach increasingly used within social and biological sciences. Within psychology in particular the term refers to an approach which combines two common uses of the term "function". In the first a behaviour or phenomenon is considered in the light of the purpose it serves for the behavioural system as a whole. Thus for one individual, aggressive behaviour may serve the function of obtaining status within a group. An example would be the football fan whose status amongst friends improved as a result of some aggressive incident.

A second, more formal, use of the term function in functional analysis refers to the description of the kind of way in which certain things relate to the problem in question. Thus it would be misleading to describe, say, alcohol as "causing" aggressive behaviour, since the research suggests a complex relationship between aggression and alcohol. For various reasons it is advantageous to describe the level of aggression as being related to alcohol (amongst other things). Borrowing from the world of mathematics and physics, the term "function" has been used to describe such a relationship, e.g. level of aggression can be seen as being, under some circumstances, a function of the intake of alcohol.

The methods of functional analysis have been used both in the study of individual cases (see e.g. Owens and Ashcroft 1982) and a range of clinical problems (see e.g. Slade 1982, Ferster 1967). The beginnings of a functional analysis of aggression have been presented elsewhere (Owens and Bagshaw 1984).

FUNCTIONAL ANALYSIS AND AGGRESSION

In the behavioural sciences, functional analysis combines both of the emphases mentioned above. To the extent that it attempts to specify the detailed form of the relationship between certain factors and a behaviour it reflects the use from mathematics and physics. Beyond this, however, it also looks at the way in which a phenomenon like aggression contributes to the system as a whole, thus reflecting the use of functional analysis in biology, anthropology etc. With respect to aggression, the notion of a functional analysis involves specifying the kinds of factors which may be implicated together with, as far as possible, a specification of the precise way in which such factors actually relate to the aggression.

As a starting point in the functional analysis of aggression, it is worth noting that two quite distinct processes may be identified which lead to aggression. These are the reactive and operant processes described in Chapter Five. Either of these is capable of producing aggression without help from any other factors and in this sense they may be regarded as fairly basic processes. The task of integration is then to outline how these basic processes may be influenced by variables identified by psychology, biology, anthropology etc.

PSYCHOLOGICAL INFLUENCES ON BASIC PROCESSES

Perhaps the most obvious influence of psychological factors on basic processes comes from the influence the two processes have on each other. Thus we have already seen how in territorial aggression behaviour which is elicited by a reactive process may later be maintained by operant reinforcement. In a similar way operant aggression may later affect reactive processes. Knutson et al. (1980) for example showed that reactive aggression could be made more likely following a history of reinforced aggression.

In addition it is clear that stimuli which indicate a particular likelihood of reinforcement will become discriminative for operant aggression. The reinforcing and punishing consequences of aggression thus have two effects on the likelihood of aggression; besides acting directly they also have an influence through the operation of discriminative stimuli.

Each of these processes may be influenced in complex ways by various other factors. The role of the social group in providing a rich potential source of reinforcers and punishers has already been noted, together with the fact that the group may influence the role of existing factors. Thus to the extent that self-control of aggression involves self-punishment, through feelings of guilt etc., it may be attenuated when a social group permits its members to diffuse the blame to the group as a whole rather than the individual. Similarly self-defined discriminative stimuli like one's own views of right and wrong may be overwhelmed by the competing effect of other stimuli provided by the remainder of the group. Finally of course the role of such factors as 'overcontrol' in the individual's history will give rise to each person having a unique history of reinforcement and punishment with often a quite idiosyncratic relationship between stimuli and behaviour. Since the reinforcers, punishers and discriminative stimuli are potentially specific to the individual, it is perhaps unsurprising that some individuals behave in a manner which seems unusual or even bizarre.

BIOLOGICAL FACTORS

As discussed in Chapter Three, the role of biological factors in aggression remains obscure. Potentially however we can note the possibility of their influence in a number of ways. Most particularly we may note that a number of drugs, including alcohol, may affect aggressive behaviour. Since all instances of aggression are necessarily mediated by biological processes, it seems reasonable to expect that substances known to affect such processes will be capable of affecting aggression. The influence of drugs and alcohol therefore merits further study.

DRUGS AND ALCOHOL

Inevitably research with human subjects, difficult at best in the field of aggression, is of limited scope when we come to consider the effects of drugs on aggression. Apart from mild drugs like alcohol and marijuana, it is difficult to conduct experiments investigating the role of such substances on aggression. Such research as has been done has typically been difficult to interpret, often using dependent variables which are far from satisfactory. Nevertheless it is probably possible to draw at least a few general conclusions. Thus alcohol has generally been found to act as a facilitator of aggression, although there appears to be little or no research in this field which distinguished between operant and reactive aggression: other evidence (q.v.) suggests that this may be important. More precisely alcohol appears to inhibit aggression at low doses, higher doses serving to enhance. Whilst this can be summarised in terms of a dose-effect curve for alcohol, it is perhaps interesting to consider that the different doses may operate on different processes. It is conceivable, for example, that a low dose may serve to decrease the aversiveness of eliciting stimuli thus removing reactive elements from measured aggression. More substantial doses may then provide a general disinhibition of punished behaviour, (including aggression) leading to a net increase.

The picture with respect to drugs of abuse is generally more difficult, since these substances are not usually appropriate as independent variables in human experiments. Such research is not entirely impossible, however. Marijuana, for example, has generally been found to decrease aggression, although systematic information is not available regarding such factors as dose-effect curves, or regarding the importance of specifying the type of aggression. Certainly such research commonly reports a minority of subjects for whom marijuana serves to enhance aggression, suggesting the role of as yet unspecified variables.

Research into animals is, of course, extensive, far too extensive for cover here. A mass of research has looked at the effect of various drugs in operant behaviour. For the present it seems reasonable to use such research as a basis for considering drug effects on operant aggression. Should such aggression later be shown to have properties making it pharmacologically distinct from other operant behaviours this would of course suggest caution in interpreting results from non-aggressive operant behaviour. Whilst no hard evidence is available on this point, there are plausible reasons for considering such a possibility.

Good reviews of the interactions between drugs and operant behaviour may be found in Blackman and Sanger (1978). Briefly the main impact of such research has been to emphasise the interdependence of drug effects on properties of the behaviour and its controlling schedule. Thus such factors as the rate of occurrence of a behaviour, the type of schedule according to which it is maintained, and the specific types of reinforcers and punishers involved can all contribute to determine whether a specific drug serves to enhance, inhibit or disrupt a behaviour. To this must, of course, be added pharmacological factors such as dose-effect curves and toxic and tolerance effects. With respect to aggression this implies that knowledge of how a drug will affect (operant) aggression will require a detailed specification of a large number of factors.

Turning to reactive aggression, we once again face a pharmacologically complex picture, but simplified a little by the fact that the dependent variable of interest is directly measured in such research. As with operant behaviour such factors as details of the controlling schedule can markedly influence the effect of drugs. Thus P-chlorophenylanaline appears to enhance reactive fighting when long inter-trial-intervals are used but not with short inter-trial-intervals. A recent review of drug effects on such forms of aggression (Sheard 1981) highlights, amongst the overall complexity of the subject, some of the main results of such work. These suggest that noradrenaline (NE), 5-hydroxytryptamine (5HT) and cholinergic interference can all influence reactive aggression. Results with both NE and 5HT have been conflicting, and appear to relate to the body's response to such interference. Thus chronic administration of tricyclic antidepressants and monoamine oxidase inhibitors, which prolong NE in the synapse increase reactive aggression. An increase in such aggression is also found in administration of dopamine, which lowers central NE. These apparently conflicting findings may be resolved by noting that the increase following dopamine takes some time to develop, suggesting a sensitivity of NE receptors and a subsequent effect similar to that of raised NE.

Perhaps of particular interest in the present context is the fact that drugs can have differing effects in reactive aggression and operant behaviour (and by implication operant aggression). Cocaine, for example, has been shown to disrupt reflexive aggression at doses which leave operant behaviour unaffected. Increasing the dose to one at which both operant behaviour and reactive behaviour are disrupted leads to tolerance developing when measuring the effects on reactive aggression with no evidence of tolerance as reflected in operant behaviour. If the operant behaviour used in such studies forms a suitable model for operant aggression, such results have both theoretical and practical significance. From a theoretical perspective the distinction between reactive and operant aggression is emphasised. From a practical perspective the results imply that drug treatment of aggressive behaviour should appropriately proceed only on the basis of a clear behavioural analysis of the type of aggression.

In addition it should be noted that many drugs

(and procedures like psychosurgery and brain stimulation) may affect motivational and perceptual processes. Such effects indicate other possible routes whereby biological factors may influence aggression. By influencing perceptual processes biological factors may disrupt the role of discriminative stimuli and even the role of eliciting stimuli in reactive aggression. At the very least this implies that an understanding of how any particular instance of violence will be affected by biological factors will require a detailed understanding of the role of basic processes, stimuli, reinforcers and punishers.

The situation is further complicated by the fact that not only will various biological factors influence aggressive, behaviour, so will aggressive behaviour influence the biological state of the organism. Aggressive behaviour like other kinds of behaviour, is capable of influencing such things as the body's hormonal state quite dramatically. Elias(1981), for example, found a marked change in the testosterone levels of male wrestlers before and after wrestling matches. It follows then that the role of biological factors is potentially quite complex, such factors influencing, and being influenced by, aggressive behaviour.

SOCIAL/ANTHROPOLOGICAL FACTORS

In many respects the role of social and cultural factors in aggressive behaviour can be seen as a parallel to the role of the immediate social environment (see Chapter Five). That is to say certain cultures will provide models of aggressive behaviour, reinforcement, aversive stimuli etc. In addition however the broader cultural factors influence the significance of the behaviour and its context for the individual. Thus in a culture or subculture in which violence is highly valued, the effect of being seen to be violent will be much different to one in which violence is condemned. Where the maintenance of status is important, a derogatory remark may be much more aversive than one in which criticism is welcomed.

In addition the cultural status of non-violence, the status of potential victims and so forth will all influence an individual's decision to attack. Thus evidence suggests that children may rapidly adopt sex-role stereotypes and be unlikely to step outside these. A boy, for example, may be much less likely to hit a girl than he would to hit another boy. Girls who have been exposed to cultural pressures which suggest that aggression is "unfeminine" may be much less likely to show aggression in similar circumstances.

Such factors may however also serve to heighten violence. Thus the notion of "women as property of their husband's" has been suggested as a possible basis for the frequency of physical attacks by husbands on wives. As long as the woman is seen as property of the man, he can feel justified in taking whatever action he wishes towards his own property. The problem is further exacerbated by the feeling in the past of some men that their wives should obey their every command. Not only does this imply that disobedience may become aversive, and hence capable of eliciting reactive aggression, but moreover that the enforcing of obedience through violence is likely to be reinforced. A similar process may be implicated through sexual possessiveness, and the notion that the offender in a "crime of passion" is somehow less culpable.

Cultural factors then may operate on reactive processes, determining what will be experienced as aversive, and operant processes, determining the roles of particular stimuli and reinforcers. These factors are also likely to affect such things as the individual's degree of self-control, both through effects on the perceived appropriateness and acceptability of the behaviour and on the perception of the status of the victim.

Aggressive behaviour is clearly a function of several types of variable; psychological, social, biological and so on. Moreover it must be remembered that just as each type of variable can affect aggression, it is also possible for each to affect the other; drunkenness, for example, may reduce the effect of cultural constraints on violence. For most of these variables the details of their interrelationships remain to be discovered. Nevertheless it is clear that any satisfactory approach to the understanding of violence will need to integrate information from a variety of sources. Obviously at the present state of knowledge a functional analysis of aggression can only be tentative. However it is clear that the various findings of different approaches to the study of aggression can potentially be integrated within such a framework. It is important of course to remember that such an analysis is intended to be very general, and that not all of the factors and processes will actually be involved in any particular instance of aggression. Rather the role of the general analysis is to indicate the potential involvement of various possible factors in specific episodes of violence. A specific instance of aggression will involve a subset of the various factors indicated by the functional analysis. Clearly however it is not necessary that all be implicated at any one time. Thus aggression may occur without reinforcement in a purely reactive process; biological disturbance may or may not be implicated in a particular episode; such factors as drugs or alcohol may be of major importance in one episode and totally absent from another. There is thus a distinction to be made between the general and the particular in functional analysis, in that a general analysis indicates the classes of variable which may in principle be implicated; a particular analysis indicates those which are in fact implicated in a single episode or series of episodes.

Such an analysis is important when one comes to consider definitions of aggression. A particular problem in defining aggression has been the recognition that the term is somewhat loosely used to cover a range of actual activities. In consequence definitions have suffered such problems as relying on the use of factors which are difficult or impossible to determine (e.g. intent) or which either unnecessarily limit aggression or are over-inclusive (e.g. causing physical harm). An alternative perspective is to note from a functional analysis perspective what factors may produce certain types of behaviour and then to determine in practice whether or not the factors under consideration do indeed form a subset of the general analysis. Such an approach, whilst unsatisfying to many academics, provides a perspective on aggression which is essentially practical, directing the attention of those concerned with the problem towards the factors most likely to be implicated and throwing open a number of possibilities for treatment.

PRACTICAL IMPLICATIONS

The possibility of a fully integrated model of violence has yet to be realised; it is clear however that a framework can be devised within which many of the results of various approaches can be incorporated. A combination of several approaches into a single model has a number of implications including;-

1. The role of variables from a number of different disciplines can be acknowledged by their incorporation into a single functional analysis, either of the problem of aggression as a whole or of specific instances of aggression.

2. Incorporation of several approaches into a single model permits the consideration of a number of treatment approaches and in particular the relationship of these to variables indicated by other approaches. For example biological approaches to treatment (e.g. by drugs) can be considered in the light of the numerous psychological factors which affect possible outcomes. Similarly the role of factors specified by one approach (e.g. the biological role of alcohol) can be understood in the context of factors noted by other approaches (e.g. basic psychological processes).

3. The potential complexity of an integrated model provides, at least in part, an explanation of the tremendous variability in aggressiveness throughout the world, since a variation in any one factor may have far reaching effects on total aggression. Moreover it appears that the complexity of the area in general is reflected in similar complexity at the level of the particular. Thus fully understanding any one person's aggression may involve an analysis which reveals circumstances very specific to that individual, another person's aggression being a function of quite different factors.

Chapter Seven

STRATEGIES FOR REDUCING VIOLENCE

It is clear from the material discussed in the foregoing chapters that violence is a problem, and one which potentially involves a large number of factors interacting in a complex manner. It seems logical, therefore, to look at this problem in the light of what limited information we possess and consider how best we might approach possible solutions to violence.

Of course, the ideal solution to the problem of violence lies in prevention: but whilst many have speculated on ways in which this may be achieved, we are still far from a universally agreed solution. Nevertheless such speculations raise interesting possibilities and some will be considered in Chapter Twelve

Of more immediate and pressing importance to most of us is the need to provide solutions to the violence which already surrounds us. Thus the probation officer, social worker, nurse, may have to deal with the aggressiveness of a particular individual. The judiciary and Government may wish to decide on policy strategies to reduce current levels of violence in society. Teachers may wish to take action to prevent or inhibit the development of aggressive lifestyles in children.

In many respects this problem of dealing with violence has parallels with the solution of other clinical problems, in which a range of strategies may be observed, usually falling between two extremes of approach. These two extremes may be summarised as the "technician" approach and the "problem solving" approach.

The pure technician approach to the solution of problems consists simply of recognising a problem and, without any consideration of its causes or origins, introducing some procedure (or "applying a technique") considered to be of use in dealing with this problem. Usually the problem is specified in terms of its gross physical characteristics and no attempt is made to sub-classify in terms of causal factors. Absolutely 'pure' technician approaches are rare, since there is usually some degree of lip-service to the role of causal factors, but good examples of largely technician modes of operation can be found in such diverse fields as medicine (e.g. the widespread use of minor tranquilisers without attempt to identify sources of stress), psychology and psychotherapy (e.g. the use of free-association techniques or hypnosis with all clients) and politics (e.g. the introduction of harsh judicial penalties for offenders). Whilst such approaches may refer to causal factors, these often consist of little more than post hoc justifications for applying the technique, all individuals presenting with similar problems being treated with the same technique. A problem solving approach on the other hand aims to base a solution on a detailed specific analysis of the individual problem. Such an approach may draw on procedures based on a number of perspectives, whilst a technician approach will more commonly derive techniques from just one discipline. In considering both approaches it is convenient to look at the interventions suggested by the disciplines involved.

SOCIAL/ANTHROPOLOGICAL

Inevitably, being concerned primarily with cultural effects on behaviour, anthropology has tended to be largely concerned with the solution to problems of violence in general rather than to the remediation of specific problems. Of course some efforts have been made to disrupt the cultures and subcultures associated with violence, ranging from the creation of youth clubs with the aim of interfering with street gang development to the outlawing of political groups with a violent or military element (e.g. the Irish Republican Army).

To a lesser extent however the principles involved in cultural change have been, one way or another, suggested for dealing with specific problems of violence. Thus one solution to the problem of dealing with a violent group has been to extract the most troublesome member from the remainder of the group - in effect to remove the individual from the troublesome subculture. The same principle of course is implicit in warnings to keep away from bad company. To some extent prison sentencing can be seen to serve this function, in that the culture to which an individual returns after several years of a prison sentence may well have changed in such a way as no longer to produce violent behaviour (Although few would regard this as the primary function of prison).

In general, however, anthropological approaches to the problem of violence have been concerned with the solution of societal, rather than individual violence. A number of attempts at Utopian societies have been both proposed and indeed attempted: rarely do such attempts survive for long, in particular suffering problems of instability and difficulties of surviving within a larger, different society. Nonetheless a few have managed to survive with little or no internal violence: on the other hand it must be remembered that such communities may in any case tend to attract those keen on social cooperation, making conflict in any event unlikely. The other main influences of anthropology have tended to operate through political and legal agencies.

POLITICAL AND JUDICIAL

For the most part political and judicial agencies have relied on the use of punishment as a controller of violence: typically the judiciary are responsible for meting out punishment, the political agencies for specifying the powers to be available to the judiciary.

In most judicial systems a range of punishments has been specified by the political powers, usually involving various forms of imprisonment. Although in most cases some attempt will be made to determine the form of punishment with reference to causal factors, there are nevertheless occasional attempts to apply a simple technician approach. Thus calls for the return of corporal punishment, or for the introduction of harsh detention centre regimes to give a "short sharp shock" are often made without consideration for the causes of the offence, trying to provide a remedy without an attempt at diagnosis.

Perhaps the most interesting aspect, however, of the judicial and political machinery's response to violence, has been its willingness to delegate at least some of the responsibility for action to other agencies. In particular governments have taken a number of steps to permit courts to enforce hospitalisation of at least some violent individuals. Again this shows the beginnings of moving away from a purely technician mode of operation, since the intention is that such a course of action will reflect particular causes of the violence, although paradoxically such measures are often adopted when the causes are least understood. That is to say, even the most expert of clinicians would agree that to explain violence in terms of, say, paranoid schizophrenia, is still to give only a loose explanation. Yet such an individual is much more likely to be sent to a secure hospital than one whose violence was a clearly understandable part of conducting, say, a bank robbery. With this in mind, it is perhaps appropriate to consider some of the techniques which may be offered by the biological and medical sciences.

BIOLOGICAL/MEDICAL TECHNIQUES

Whilst a number of techniques devised from physical models of aggression can be identified, the majority can be summarised under the two headings surgical and chemical. In the former we may include all those surgical procedures whose purpose is, of itself, to cure the violence. Under chemical procedures we may include not only such procedures as drug treatments but also the use of such techniques as hormone implants. (Whilst these are administered surgically, it is the hormone, not the surgery, which is presumed to have the effect: it is sensible therefore to include such procedures under the "chemical" heading.)

Surgical Procedures

A number of surgical procedures have been proposed for dealing with the problem of violence. Whilst some of these, as mentioned in Chapter 3, are actually aimed primarily at curing a disease of which the violence is a symptom (e.g. the excision of a brain tumour) others have been devised primarily with the aim of reducing the violence itself.

Perhaps the most well-known of such procedures is the prefrontal lobotomy, in which lesions are made in such a way as to isolate the frontal lobes of the brain. In fact the results of such operations have proved highly variable, both in

terms of main and side effects: in consequence some
workers (e.g. Moyer 1976) have concluded that it
should probably not be used at all for aggression
control. Similar temporal lobe surgery has also
produced a number of side effects perhaps more
severe than the original problem (Terzian and Ore
1955).

The use of amygdalectomy has been regarded as
rather more promising by some workers (e.g. Moyer
1976). Again, however, a number of side effects
have been noted including memory defects, abdominal
pain and vomiting (Şawa et. al. 1954) and a case of
diabetes insipidus (Heimburger et. al. 1966). To
what extent these and other side effects constitute
an acceptable price to pay for the increased control
of hostility is of course hard to specify. In
general it is agreed that psychosurgery, because of
its irreversibility, unreliability and risk of side
effects should be used, if at all, as a "last
resort" procedure. Even then some would regard the
procedure as unacceptable: Breggin (1972) for
example cites a number of reports of psychosurgery,
including one operation on a five-year old child in
the U.S.A. At the same time, he notes, such
procedures have been outlawed in the Soviet Union
for decades.

An alternative to the excision or lesioning of
brain structures is the electrical stimulation of
neurological structures thought to serve an
aggression-inhibiting role. Whilst such an approach
has had impressive results in animal studies, the
value of such work in controlling human aggression
has yet to be demonstrated, and many prominent
workers in this field have concluded that such
procedures will not be of practical value in solving
problems of human aggression.

Of course the brain is not the only organ to
have been subject to surgical intervention. A
number of attempts were made during the 1950's, when
hormonal explanations of behaviour were more
popular. The main effect of castration on
behaviour, however, seems to relate to sexual
arousal rather than aggressiveness. As with
psychosurgery a number of somatic complaints have
been noted as a side effect of castration, including
weight gain, deterioration in general health, and
premature signs of ageing (Bremer 1959). Again, the
problems of irreversibility and the questionable
status of "free choice" when the alternative is a
long prison sentence have made castration
unacceptable in many societies. Since its role as a

controller of aggression appears minimal, and since
many of the same chemical effects can be obtained
without castration, it seems likely to fall into
disuse.

Chemical Procedures

The use of therapeutic drugs in the treatment of
aggressive behaviour has become particularly
widespread with the growth in the use of general
psychotropic medication. In general such use
presupposes at least a minimal appreciation of the
causal processes in aggression, although the use of
powerful sedatives (e.g. sodium amytal) has been
suggested in cases of extreme emergency. In
non-emergency settings the probable causes of the
aggression can often be identified, making a more
precise approach to medication feasible. In dealing
with violence associated with psychotic states
medication will of course be concerned with the
psychosis itself as well as the control of the
aggression. In this context it has been reported
(Itil 1980) that neuroleptics which have primarily
sedative effects (e.g. chlorpromazine) have a more
rapid effect on aggressive behaviour than those
which are primarily antipsychotic (e.g.
haloperidol). Where aggressive behaviour has been
suspected of association with epileptic disorder,
however, increased aggressiveness has been
associated with increased use of anticonvulsant
(e.g. Landholt 1960). For problems of intermittent
or isolated aggressive outbursts benzodiazepines
(e.g. Ativan) have been suggested. Such compounds
have also been proposed for the control of
aggression associated with withdrawal from drug
abuse (Itil 1981). In general drug therapy has been
seen as treating not aggression itself, but rather
psychiatric problems believed to be associated with
the aggression.

Inevitably such an approach also has its
problems. The difficulties of fitting drug
treatment to aggressive behaviour without careful
specification of the underlying process have been
mentioned earlier (e.g. Chapter Six). In addition a
number of unacceptable side effects have been
reported with many of the drugs used;
chlorpromazine, for example, has been associated
with hypertension on rapid or repeated use (Kline
and Angst 1975). Ethical disquiet may also arise
with respect to drug treatments, in particular where
these are suggested for highly vulnerable groups

like children and the mentally handicapped.

Further problems may arise from the properties of the drugs themselves. The benzodiazepines, for example, are now generally agreed to be of value in short term use only, and the Committee on Safety of Medicines has discouraged prescribing for any longer period than a matter of weeks: besides ineffectiveness, such drugs carry the possibility of establishing dependence with long term use. Whilst drug treatments will undoubtedly continue to play a part in the management of aggression, therefore, it would be naive to think of them providing a completely effective or satisfactory solution in the immediate future.

Psychological procedures

Recent years have seen the application of a number of psychological procedures to the problems of violent behaviour. Sometimes the procedures used have been specially devised for the treatment of violent behaviour. Often however the procedures are adaptations of those already used for the treatment of other psychological difficulties. In particular the general group of procedures known as "Behaviour Modification" have been variously applied to dealing with violence. Thus Pinkston et al. (1973) report the use of an extinction procedure with a three and a half year old boy. Observation of the child's frequent aggressive episodes led to the suspicion that much of the reinforcement for such behaviour came from the teachers, who responded to the outbursts either by reprimands or attempts to reason with the child. By instructing the teachers to cease giving attention in response to aggressive episodes Pinkston et al. were able to decrease the amount of the child's time spent being aggressive from an original level of almost 30% to a level close to zero. This type of procedure, the removal of reinforcers which currently serve to maintain the behaviour, has been demonstrated to be effective in a substantial number of cases (e.g. Madsen et al. 1968: Ward and Baker 1968). It depends of course on successful identification of the reinforcers, and to the extent that this constitutes (at least in part) an individual analysis of the problem may relate more closely to "problem solving" rather than "technician approaches".

Such a procedure is however, of limited applicability. It requires correct identification of the reinforcers, control of the reinforcers, and also requires that the aggressive behaviour be of such a quality that it can safely be ignored. These factors will not always apply. Thus the behaviour of a bully in a school playground may be reinforced by the behaviour of the victim, or the behaviour of a peer group. In many such cases the therapist will be unable or unwilling to affect these reinforcers and it will not be possible to implement the procedure.

Even where control of the reinforcers is possible, it may not always be possible or desirable to implement the procedure. Thus, if the extinction procedure requires that the aggressive behaviour be ignored, it may be inappropriate to implement the procedure because of the risk of serious harm: it is one thing to ignore a kick delivered by a small child, quite a different thing to ignore one delivered by a fully developed large adult. Extinction procedures do not bring about an immediate decrease in aggression: the decrease is typically gradual and it may be days or weeks before the aggression is completely eliminated. To ignore aggressive behaviour for such a period will often be impractical.

An additional problem is raised by the very nature of extinction schedules. Considerable research, and much clinical experience, show that the initial effect of an extinction programme may be an intensification, rather than a decrease, of the behaviour in question. Whilst such an intensification is only temporary, it can exacerbate the problem of using extinction programmes.

Nevertheless there are clearly a number of situations in which such a procedure could be of value. Where an extinction schedule is to be implemented, the following should always occur:-

(a) An initial assessment of the extent of the violence prior to extinction. This assessment may be of the frequency of violent outbursts, their duration, their severity or any other measure which is both appropriate and susceptible to reliable measurement. By obtaining such information both before and during the intervention process it is possible to detect early signs of change in the level of aggression. Such early signs may be too slight to be noticed by casual observation yet provide valuable information regarding such things as whether reinforcers have been correctly identified.

(b) Every possible step should be taken to ensure that the behaviour is no longer reinforced.

Thus in an institutional setting it may be necessary to instruct all staff who interact with the individual, whether as a professional involvement (e.g. nurses, social workers) or not (e.g. ward cleaners).

(c) Similarly all those involved in the programme should be warned of the possibility of a temporary intensification of the problem, and reassured that this will indeed pass.

(d) Where possible every effort should be made to "shift" the reinforcement the individual is to lose to some other, more positive behaviour. Ideally the alternative behaviour selected should be incompatible with the violent behaviour. Not only is it ethically desirable that existing levels of reinforcement be maintained: such procedures also enhance the possibility of a successful intervention, besides providing an opportunity to introduce useful rehabilitative programmes.

Related to the use of extinction programmes is the use of punishment procedures. Punishment alone has of course obvious problems in dealing with aggressive behaviour, since punishment of operant aggression may provide an aversive stimulus which gives rise to reactive aggression. Nonetheless careful use of punishment has provided the basis for intervention in some cases. In a widely reported series of studies in "Achievement Place", a home for delinquent boys, Phillips (1968) reported a number of successes in modifying undesirable behaviour. In one such programme the boys earned points, (exchangeable for such things as time spent watching T.V.), episodes of aggressiveness leading to loss of these points. Measurements of rates of aggressiveness before and after the introduction of the procedure showed a rapid reduction in aggressive behaviour.

Such a procedure is however far from universally effective. The prison system in the United Kingdom for example operates an analogous system in the use of remission. A prisoner can normally expect to be discharged before the specified term of the sentence, with, normally up to one-third of the sentence being remitted. Such remission will normally be lost, in part or in total, if the individual offends against the prison discipline, e.g. by fighting, assaulting prison officers etc. Such a system has obvious parallels with the Achievement Place system, yet assaults continue to occur in prisons with alarming frequency. The reasons for this lack of effectiveness are far from clear but may relate to the nature of the aggression (the Phillips study was concerned primarily with threats and similar verbal aggression), with the amount of reinforcements available (reinforcement of aggression in a U.K. prison may be stronger than the reinforcement of threats in a U.S. delinquent home) or both. It may of course be the case that the two behaviours represent different types of aggression, the aggression in Achievement Place being largely operant, that in prisons being largely reactive.

In general it appears to be the case that punishment is most effective when combined with an extinction programme. In the elimination of a large number of types of undesirable behaviour a procedure known as "Time Out From Reinforcement" (usually shortened to Time Out or TO) has had some effectiveness. The procedure involves responding to an aggressive episode by instituting conditions where not only will the behaviour not be reinforced, but the opportunity to earn reinforcement for other behaviours is also, for a time, lost. Typically this involves removal of the individual to a place where she/he can be left alone for a brief period, such as an empty room. Thus Clark et al (1973) used a TO procedure in the elimination of aggressive behaviour by an eight year old mentally handicapped chld. Treatment consisted of three of more minutes of TO whenever an attack occured. By sequentially applying the procedure to the child's different types of aggressive behaviour (against people, against property etc.) Clark et al. were able not only to reduce the level of aggression almost to zero but were also able clearly to demonstrate that it was indeed the TO which was responsible. Similar results have been reported by a number of other workers (e.g. Patterson, Cobb and Ray 1973; Drabman and Spitalnick 1973).

The use of TO is not however without its problems. In general it is agreed that TO is most likely to be effective when used in conjunction with reinforcement of appropriate behaviours. This of course highlights one of the greatest problems of TO, that of determining the duration of TO periods. Since any form of rehabilitation is to all intents and purposes impossible without reinforcement, each minute spent in TO is a minute's potential rehabilitation lost. Moreover the longer an individual remains in TO the greater the risk of actually exhibiting some appropriate behaviour which will remain unreinforced and thereby possibly more difficult to obtain later. In general most studies have used TO periods either of the order of 2-3 minutes in total or alternatively have involved observing the individual in TO and returning them to their normal surroundings within a minute or so of their becoming calm. Occasionally such short periods may necessitate the individual being returned to TO within a short time followng a second aggressive outburst. This appears to happen infrequently, however, and when it does happen seems to be only a temporary phase. As a result it is generally agreed that the duration of TO should be as short as possible and that the individual should not be kept in TO for more than one or two minutes following the disappearance of the problem behaviour.

Inevitably such procedures as extinction and punishment are largely if not exclusively directed at operant aggression. Much human aggression, however, appears to be primarily reactive, necessitating a somewhat different approach.

The treatment of reactive aggression is primarily directed at teaching an alternative response to the stimulation prompting the reactive aggression. Carr and Binkoff (1982) describe the use of systematic desensitisation in eliminating reactive aggression. Such a procedure involves several stages. First the individual is taught some response which is incompatible with aggression: most commonly the procedure taught is that of progressive muscle relaxation, based on the method of Jacobsen (1938). Having been taught such a response the individual can then learn to use this as an alternative to aggression in progressively more difficult situations. This involves the preparation of a hierarchy of such problems, the individual specifying and ordering a range of problems from those which could be coped with easily to those which would involve great difficulty. These are then presented successively, a more difficult item only being approached once the easier items have been managed. Thus in Carr and Binkoff's example the first step was to teach relaxation. Once relaxation could be achieved with ease, a hierarchy of difficult situations concerned with "disrespect from others" was constructed. The client was then asked to imagine the easiest of the situations listed and to relax whilst doing so: once relaxation in response to imagining the easiest situation was mastered, the next situation was presented and relaxation learned as a response to this. The procedure then continues in the same way until the whole hierarchy has been mastered. Of course the hierarchies themselves will be specific to individual clients, implying at least a partial analysis of the aggression and, again, moving away from a purely "technician" level of operation. Similarly a number of variations on the basic procedure may be employed. In most cases the learning of a relaxation response to imagined problems will be followed by a period of learning to relax in progressively more difficult "real" situations: in some circumstances the use of imagination may be omitted and training began directly with real problems. Other responses may also be used: Smith (1973) for example reports the use of laughter as a response incompatible with aggression.

The value of systematic desensitisation in the control of aggression is indicated by a number of studies (e.g. Evans 1970, Rimm et al. 1971). In general however such a procedure is used in conjunction with other procedures in order to maximise the probability of linking a response other than aggression to the problem situation(s).

One such procedure derives from the Rational Emotive Therapy (RET) of Ellis (1962). In this the irrational thoughts held by an individual are confronted directly and replaced by more rational alernatives. Thus the individual who responds to a critical comment by thinking "this person's trying to make me look small", with consequent aggression, may be taught to think along the lines "this person has seen a mistake I've made and feels obliged to point it out, not realising that I'll thereby lose status in the eyes of the people around" or "O.K., so I've made a mistake, but the people around me will accept that, they don't expect me to be 100% perfect". By replacing irrational, aversive thoughts with thoughts which are more rational and more neutral the individual can learn to respond in a more calm and realistic manner. Most of the application of RET has been outside the context of aggression, but occasional reports of the application of RET to problems of aggressiveness appear (e.g. Di Giuseppe 1977). Application of RET typically involves a number of stages. In the first of these the therapist explains to the client the reasoning behind the therapy, that the content of (often irrational) thoughts can have a marked influence on behaviour. In the next stage the therapist and the client work together to identify irrational thoughts and beliefs which are causing problems. Thus if a client acts in accordance with a belief that "unless I can dominate all the people around me I won't be respected" such a belief can be challenged and replaced with some more realistic perception of the world. It is important to note that such beliefs may not have been explicitly spelled out by the client before the commencement of therapy, but may rather be implicit in the way they behave. Challenging of irrational beliefs may involve the discussing of evidence which contradicts the belief, identification of inconsistencies, or the presentation of the beliefs to the client by the therapist, the client then being asked to argue against the beliefs. Thus in the example above the therapist might point out occasions where the client was unable to be dominant yet still earned considerable respect: or the therapist may point out that many members of the social group are respected even though only one can be the dominant member: or the therapist may play the part of the client, presenting the belief in such a way that the client can detect its flaws and argue against it. In the final stages of therapy the client is encouraged to identify irrational thoughts in everyday life and to generate rational alternatives. It would appear that the main role of RET is in dealing with reactive aggression, although it will of course also have a role where the individual holds irrational beliefs regarding aggressive behaviour and subsequent reinforcement.

A further strategy also involves the changing of the individual's response to situations, but with clear relevance to both reactive and operant aggression. This is the procedure known as assertiveness training. Workers using this approach distinguish strictly between assertiveness and aggression, pointing out that not only is skilled assertiveness a positive advantage, where aggressiveness can be a disadvantage, but also that in some cases a total lack of assertiveness may eventually result in a totally unacceptable level of aggression (as in the studies of the overcontrolled personality see Chapter Six).

In assertiveness training a number of procedures are used to teach the client to behave in a way which will obtain the required goals without generating hostility or some other undesirable consequence from others. Important here is the concept of the "minimal effective response", i.e. that response which will achieve the desired goal with minimal effort and least risk of generating hostility in others. At the same time the client is encouraged to ientify with the needs and rights of the other person. In this way the client can learn to be assertive and obtain desired goals whilst at the same time minimising the risk of antagonising others. Of course the response selected will not always be successful, and it will usually be necessary to teach the client to gradually escalate the assertiveness when necessary.

In practice such procedures involve the therapist and client both identifying areas where appropriate assertiveness needs to be learned, identifying the client's normal pattern of response to such situations and the consequences of such responses. Alternative, assertive responses are then explored and practised both with the therapist and in the actual situations. As with RET it is not unusual for the therapist to role play the part of the client, the client taking the role of some individual who may be difficult to deal with.

A number of studies point to the value of assertiveness training in dealing with aggressive behaviour (e.g. Wallace et al. 1973, Foy et al. 1975). Typically such training has been used with individuals who behave in an "overcontrolled" manner, teaching them to be assertive and prevent situations developing where their control is no longer sufficient. A few points are however worth noting regarding assertiveness training. Although a number of procedures have been used to teach assertive responses there does not appear to be any unequivocal "best" way. Gradual shaping through successive approximations to the desired behaviour, instruction, modelling of the behaviour by the therapist, role play and video feedback have all been used with success, and it seems likely that in most cases a combination of these will be maximally effective. The "best" way of teaching in any particular situation is likely to be a function of, at least, the characteristics of the client, of the problem, and of the others involved in the problem.

It is also important to note that studies have, in general, found assertion to be often quite situation-specific. That is to say the individual may have no difficulty being assertive in one setting (e.g. at work or in the therapist's office) but may have considerable difficulty in other settings (e.g. when at home or with friends). Correspondingly the assertion learned during assertion training may also be situation-specific. It is therefore important to take positive steps to cover a wide range of situations in training, and to encourage the client to recognise as many as possible of the potential applications of assertiveness training in day-to-day life.

Similar issues arise in a related approach to dealing with the problem of aggression, that of Social Skills Training (SST): indeed assertiveness training may be considered a subset of general social skills and hence an appropriate component in SST programmes. SST aims to teach a range of skills in which the individual may be lacking and which relate to social behaviour. Such training is relevant to problems of aggression to the extent that the individual's aggressive behaviour results from inadequate social skills. Thus the individual who is unable to relate positively to a social group may find that the only strategy available for acceptance with the group consists of aggressive behaviour: such an individual does not know any other way to gain acceptance, and the grudging acceptance obtained may be preferable to social isolation. Or the individual may be completely unable to relate to others, resulting in the presence of others being seen as aversive and hence producing reactive aggression. As with assertiveness training a range of teaching procedures may be used to obtain the desired skills, and as with all the procedures discussed careful monitoring is important in order to identify rapidly the success (or otherwise) of intervention programmes. Many SST programmes operate as group programmes, with several clients collaborating in role plays, discussions etc. Although its use extends considerably beyond problems of aggression, there do exist reports of its successful use with violent individuals.

Inevitably it is not possible here to describe exhaustively all the methods that psychology has developed for the control of aggression. Further approaches to the control of aggressive behaviour include "Problem Solving Training" (discussed in detail by Goldstein 1982) and the use of self-control skills (presented in a variety of contexts by Thorsen and Mahoney 1968). A number of attempts have also been made to combine the various techniques into "packages" or combinations of procedures. One such package for the treatment of reactive aggression has been described by Novaco (1975). Clients in such programmes are presented with a range of alternative responses to stressful situations in order to replace the aggression that such situations normally elicit. Included in such packages may be relaxation training, assertion and RET-type cognitive treatments. Such packages have been used successfully with a number of violence-related problems including child abuse, aggression by those in authority (e.g. businessmen, police officers, etc.) and the treatment of violent offenders.

It is clear, then, that there exist a number of potentially useful techniques for the control of violent behaviour. Although few of these achieve the purely "technician" approach where treatment is determined by identification rather than analysis of the problem the level of analysis required may be minimal, often consisting of little more than identifying the aggression as either operant (e.g. extinction procedures) or reactive (e.g. the Novaco package). Results from a number of studies suggest that considerable success may be obtained with such an approach, the intervention being sufficiently closely matched to the initial problem for the procedure to work.

In some cases, however, the use of such a straightforward approach may obtain less success than would have been hoped, or indeed no success at all. Such failure may have a number of reasons. The type of aggression (reactive or operant) may not have been correctly identified. There may be other factors which interfere with the treatment programme (e.g. resentment towards the therapist). Or it may not be possible to control those factors (e.g. suspected sources of reinforcement) believed to be implicated in the violent behaviour. Under such circumstances it may be necessary to produce a "customised" intervention rather than a straightforward "package". The production of such a custom-made treatment programme requires a detailed analysis of all available information relevant to the problem, the integration of such information into a coherent model or theory of the processes involved, and the devising of a suitable intervention.

The use of such an approach ("Problem Solving" rather than "technician") has developed in parallel with the functional analysis perspective described in Chapter Six and in a sense represents the use of such an approach not to a general problem (like violence) but to a specific problem (a particular individual's violence). Detailed analyses of one individual's violence is likely to highlight a number of specific features particular to the person in question. Whilst this implies that, to some extent, each individual must be approached anew, it is nevertheless possible to note some general features of the problem solving approach which will apply in most if not all cases.

The first stage in producing a formulation of how various factors combine to produce a particular individual's violent behaviour is obviously to obtain as much as possible of the information which may be relevant. For convenience a tendency has developed amongst those working within this approach to classify information into what has become known as the "ABC" framework. Here A stands for Antecedents, B for the Behaviour, and C for the Consequences. That is to say, as much relevant information as possible is obtained about what led up to a violent episode, what form it took, and what the consequences of the violence were. This then provides clues as to what extent reactive and operant processes were operating, together with an indication of other possible contributory factors. At this stage it is also important to obtain information regarding the "baseline" aggression, that is to say its frequency, intensity etc., prior to starting intervention.

The second stage involves integrating this information in such a way as to provide a provisional explanation of the behaviour: such an explanation will usually provide an indication of suitable interventions. Thus one individual seen by the first author became very self-critical after aggressive outbursts, feeling guilty about the violence that had been shown. This led to depression and associated apathy, making it difficult to introduce any procedure aimed directly at the violent behaviour. By dealing first with the depression and self-condemnation it was possible later to look at the factors associated with aggression and to introduce programmes aimed at reduction. Attempts to introduce such programmes directly would have met with little enthusiasm and been unlikely to succeed.

The third stage, to some extent going on at the same time as the second stage, involves the evaluation of the intervention. By comparing such measures as the frequency of violent behaviour before and after intervention it is possible to assess whether a programme is in fact working. If a programme fails to work when the formulation says that it should, it follows that the formulation must be wrong. A new formulation must therefore be drawn

up in the light of the additional information which
has become available. This revised formulation then
forms the basis for a further intervention programme
and the process repeated from the second stage. In
this way each successive intervention provides more
and more information, enabling better and better
formulations and progresssively increasing the
chances of success.

A number of issues arise from the use of such an
approach. Correct identification of the relevant
variables permits not only the design of an
intervention but also direct assessment of the long
term outcome in terms of the extent to which the
intervention brings about temporary or permanent
change in important variables. Thus if an
individual's violence within an institution leads
them to obtain more attention from the institution
staff, the long term outcome of changing staff
behaviour (and hence eliminating the reinforcement
of violence) will depend upon (a) whether the staff
continue in their new pattern of behaviour, which
will usually involve both failing to reinforce the
violence AND explicitly reinforcing some alternative
behaviour (b) whether or not provision is made to
ensure that any new staff also behave appropriately
and (c) whether or not the social environment in any
new setting (to which the individual may later move)
also maintains the programme.

One of the implications of this is that a
successful programme will need to distinguish what
has been called arbitrary and natural reinforcement.
The latter are those reinforcements which naturally
maintain behaviour in society: a friendly greeting
in response to a "Good morning" for example.
Arbitrary reinforcements are those which bear no
natural relationship to the behaviour, for example
the giving of sweets to an aggressive child in order
to reinforce non-violent play. Whilst a programme
may use arbitrary reinforcement to establish a new
pattern of behaviour, a well-designed programme will
arrange an eventual transition from arbitrary to
natural reinforcement. Usually this will involve
the gradual fading out of arbitrary reinforcement
until control of the behaviour has transferred to
natural reinforcers. Whilst this may eventually
give the impression that the behaviour is being
maintained without any reinforcement there is in
fact no experimental evidence to show that this is
in fact possible, and in such circumstances it seems
rather to be the case that the natural reinforcers
have "taken over" from the arbitrary ones.

A further point of relevance is that it may often be appropriate to produce not only a formulation of the factors maintaining the behaviour, but also of those which gave rise to the behaviour in the first place. If this is not done there remains the risk that the combination of circumstances which originally produced the violence may recur, producing the violent behaviour again and resulting in the intervention having only a temporary effect. Associated with this is the importance of identifying similarities and differences in an individual's episodes of aggression. An individual in the community may, for example, show a high degree of reactive aggression as a result of inability to relate to family, workmates etc. Placed in an institution, such circumstances may not occur, producing an immediate elimination of this (reactive) aggression. Such an individual, however, may by this time be a highly skilled aggressor and find that continued aggression leads to increased status, power etc. (Operant aggression). The appearance would be that of an individual whose aggression had remained the same outside and inside the institution. Programmes successful at eliminating the (operant) aggression within the institution, however, may result in little or no change in the (reactive) aggression occurring outside. The individual may thus be seen by the institution as one whose aggression has been successfully treated and therefore discharged. Yet the treatment programme, whilst dealing successfully with the violence within the institution, may have left violence outside the institution totally unaffected.

It is therefore of particular importance to gather information not only about current violence but also, if possible, about past violence, in order to detect any changes in the controlling conditions. It is moreover important to be cautious when any change in environment is planned: the more substantial the change, the more important the caution. At all times it is important to note that behaviour change involves a change in the relationship between the individual and the environment: such a change in one setting will not necessarily extend to other settings without careful programming.

Inevitably, since each intervention will depend upon the individual formulation, it is not possible to give details on how such interventions should proceed. In general terms however three principles

111

have proved of wide applicability in devising
intervention strategies: these are the principles
of Elimination, Amelioration and Compensation. That
is to say as far as possible factors which maintain
the aggression should be eliminated, either by
making sure that they do not physically occur, or by
arranging that when they do occur they no longer
have the same function. Thus in the first case it
may be possible to arrange the environment in such a
way that the factor no longer occurs: in an
institution, for example, two individuals may be
sufficiently aversive to each other as to produce
rapid reactive aggression whenever they meet. By
moving one of them to another part of the
institution such violence can be avoided. A second
way to eliminate the problem, however, might be not
to separate the two but to take positive action to
help them resolve their differences and, if not
actually become friends, at least to tolerate each
others' presence. In this way the variable would be
functionally eliminated without actually being
physically eliminated.

In many cases, of course, relevant variables
will not be completely under control, and rather
than completely eliminating a factor it may only be
possible to reduce or ameliorate its effects. Thus
it may not be possible to totally ignore violent
behaviour by an individual whose violence is
reinforced by the attention: nevertheless it is
possible to arrange that only minimal attention is
given. Thus in one case presented to the first
author a resident in a home for the mentally
handicapped broke windows in the institution, such
behaviour apparently being reinforced by the
considerable fuss which ensued. Whilst such
behaviour could not be completely ignored, it proved
possible to clean and dress the resulting cuts with
a minimum of fuss, reducing the total reinforcement
and thus contributing to the elimination of the
behaviour.

The third process, that of compensation, should
be considered parallel to, rather than as an
alternative to, the principles of elimination and
amelioration. The aim here is to ensure that action
is taken in a programme to compensate both for
factors which serve to maintain aggression and,
where appropriate, to compensate for loss of such
things as reinforcement as part of an overall
programme. Thus the individual whose aggression is
reinforced by the status it provides within a social
group should be taught other ways of gaining such

status in order to compensate for any loss of status that might accrue from reduced aggression. Without such compensation there is always a risk that the individual will conclude that the change has been too costly and will revert to the original behaviour. Even where it has been possible to eliminate successfully such things as reinforcement, compensation will still enhance success. Without such compensation there remains the danger that the individual will persist in the behaviour despite it no longer being successful, since it still remains the only behaviour ever experienced as successful. Until an alternative is provided the individual may remain remarkably persistent in attempting to obtain reinforcemnt through the previously successful aggression.

Finally it is important to note that in drawing out the links between various factors a number of these will "feed back" into each other producing a so-called "vicious circle". Such points in the process often represent points of particular importance for intervention, as these will otherwise tend rapidly to re-stabilise following intervention. For example one such circle might involve an individual who is aggressive towards others and is thereby rejected: the rejection produces further rejection and so on. Obviously any attempt to eliminate the aggressive behaviour will be well advised to attempt to disrupt such a vicious circle.

DEALING WITH VIOLENT INCIDENTS

Whilst prevention of violent incidents is desirable it will often be the case that workers in the caring professions are confronted either with violence or the imminent threat of violence. Such violence may occur in the doctor's surgery, the hospital ward, the prison wing and so on. It will be clear from earlier discussion of the causes of violence that such incidents are potentially very complex and that rigid guidelines are inappropriate in advising how best to deal with such problems.

Nevertheless it is possible to consider violent incidents in the context of what is known about the processes involved and thereby to note at least some of the issues which may be relevant. Inevitably selecting an appropriate course of action when confronted with a violent incident is easiest when the factors involved are well understood. If for example reactive processes can be seen to be at work, it may be possible to remove the aversive stimuli to which the individual is reacting. Besides aspects of the social and physical environment it is important to note that aspects of behaviour may be aversive and give rise to reactive aggression. Thus speaking to an angry person in a hostile, aggressive or even patronising manner may be sufficient to trigger an attack. Moreover it is important to note that the triggering events may be quite specific to each individual; on one occasion for example the first author was attacked after smiling at a psychiatric patient on entering. For this particular patient smiling obviously had particular connotations resulting in an aggressive outburst.

Similarly with respect to operant aggression it is possible to note a few relevant issues. Obviously it is not normally a good idea to reinforce aggressive behaviour. Again, however, it is important to note that reinforcers may be idiosyncratic. Thus a threatening response to an aggressive act may in fact serve to reinforce such aggression, making it more likely to recur. If the aim of the original act was to disturb or distress the person at whom it was directed signs of such disturbance serve to indicate that the action was successful.

On the other hand it is clear that totally ignoring the early stages of aggression may be equally harmful. It was noted above that extinction procedures could often give rise to, in the short term, increased levels of aggression. If the individual has a history of successful violence, to be ignored may result in escalation of the action. In both this context, and the context of reactive aggression, the strategy most likely to be successful is one of "calm normality". That is to say the response given should be as close as possible to normal interpersonal behaviour. A calm, confident and reasonable reaction to the initial signs of violence may permit a potentially explosive situation to be defused.

Under ideal circumstances it may be possible to take further measures to handle violent situations. Often for example it will be possible to indicate that an attack has little chance of succeeding. This may involve a range of strategies including not turning one's back on an aggressor unneccesarily (since this would indicate increased probability of the attack succeeding) and ensuring that sufficient support (in the form of additional colleagues etc.)

is available to indicate that an attack will not succeed. Such measures of course operate by manipulating the discriminative stimuli of which aggression is a function and thus reducing its probability.

Because of the rich variety of human behaviour, and the number of ways in which people may respond to what goes on around them it is not possible to give rigid guides on how to behave in an aggressive incident. What defuses one situation may cause another to flare up. Nevertheless a few basic principles will be of value in the majority of situations. Such principles include:

1. Acting calmly. An emotional or aggressive response to a disturbed individual is much more likely to reinforce the person's aggression, to elicit reactive aggression, or both. Whilst it is rarely possible to know all the potential reinforcers and triggers for aggression, the kinds of behaviour which a person normally encounters without becoming violent will usually be fairly safe.

2. Avoiding any behaviour which increases the chance of an attack succeeding. At its most obvious level this may mean avoiding giving an aggressive individual a weapon, or avoiding turning one's back on such a person. This may not be as straightforward as first appears. Giving someone a cup of tea may set the occasion for friendly rather than hostile interaction; but a hot liquid may also constitute a particularly vicious weapon.

3. Observing the progress of the aggression. Few aggressive incidents occur instantaneously. More commonly escalation proceeds through a number of stages. By noting whether an individual becomes more or less agitated, tense or aggressive, it is often possible to identify more precisely those actions which serve to calm and those which serve to inflame.

4. Attempt to relax the aggressive individual. To be in the presence of a tense person often creates tension in others. Calming an aggressive person, correspondingly, involves remaining calm oneself. Workers likely to be confronted with violence should ensure that they are adequately prepared for such events, retaining a calm an unruffled manner and attempting to induce similar calmness in the aggressor. Encouraging the aggressor to sit down may be sufficient to delay or divert the possibility of attack. If such an individual can be seated, the person dealing with

115

the incident will normally sit down as well; ideally the two will sit somewhat to the side of each other, presenting the least effective position for a target.

Such strategies are of course of value only in the short term and should be regarded as interim "holding" measures in dealing with violence rather than as solutions. When a situation has been calmed in this way the major part of the work remains to be done. Violent or near-violent incidents should always be investigated in detail, covering such issues as (a) what signs might have enabled the violence to be better predicted (b) what changes in strategy might have led to a more satisfactory outcome (c) what changes in routine might help prevent or deal with such problems and (d) what steps should be taken to help those at whom the violence was directed? With respect to the latter point it is important to note the variety of emotional responses which may result from being the target of an attack: besides responses like fear and anxiety, other responses like guilt and denial have been reported.

In general the caring professions have taken considerable interest in methods of dealing with violent attacks. There has usually been little support for the teaching of complex self defence skills, not only because the main aim of training is seen as prevention but also because of their frequent impracticality. Most care agents would be reluctant to use, say, karate techniques against their clientele because of the difficulty of avoiding serious harm. Other martial arts procedures like aikido and judo may provide a finer degree of control but typically require years of dedicated training. Moreover such procedures may be limited in their applicability in settings like confined, cluttered spaces and will often involve the trainee in considerably more harm and injury during training than would be experienced in a professional lifetime of risk of attack. (The first author, a black belt judo international, suffered numerous injuries in a ten year period including a broken ankle, a dislocated collarbone, chipped teeth, a cauliflower ear and a bent nose. Few people experience a fraction of these injuries as a result of personal attack.) The teaching of such skills, then, is usefully limited to a few simple procedures which can be safely practised. Whilst this gives only limited skill it is probably as much as is appropriate for most workers. A number of such procedures have been outlined elsewhere (see e.g. French 1983 pp. 249ff). Further discussion of aggression management within a specifically nursing context may be found in Dingwall (1984), Gibbs (1984) and Orr (1984).

Whilst systematic research on the effectiveness of different strategies is rare, much can be learned from those who interact frequently with potentially violent individuals who frequently report on approaches which have been found useful in practice (see e.g. Packham 1978, Carney 1979, Leiba 1980). Professionals working in settings where violence is a possibility should ensure that they are familiar with their employer's code of practice, that necessary facilities and resources (e.g. alarm bells, support staff) are available and that their colleagues are similarly aware of the relevant issues. For those closely involved with violent or potentially violent individuals specific training schemes are available. The English National Board, for example, operates a post-qualification course (ENB course 955) which, whilst primarily aimed at the nursing profession, is open and of value to most professionals. Wherever possible, organisations dealing with violent individuals should ensure that training of this or a similar kind is available.

CONCLUSION

Clearly each perspective which has come to deal with the problem of violence has provided prospective solutions. To some extent the type of solution appropriate will depend on the type of aggression: social and judicial solutions to social violence, medical solutions to those caused by medical problems, psychological solutions to psychological causes etc. An obvious implication of this is that the violence needs to be clearly understood before committing oneself to a particular type of solution. The issue can be seen to extend beyond these demarcation limits however. Thus social and political change can affect psychological processes: for example the cultures in which violence is unacceptable (Chapter Four) are, because of this, ones in which less reinforcement is available for aggressive behaviour. Similarly the interrelationship of the physiological and the behavioural (Chapter Three) suggests that both may have a part to play in the solution of problems of violence. For example pharmacological intervention may produce a rapid decrease in aggressiveness, but suffer from unwanted side effects (e.g. general sedation) and be only temporary until the body has reacted to the chemical disturbances. Psychological approaches, less likely to have side effects and more likely to be slow-acting, may on occasion need to be combined with physical treatment in order to produce short-term control until the psychological procedures take effect. Such strategies call for close collaboration between professionals: many drugs will interfere with the individual's learning capacity, calling for such things as progressive reductions in dosage as the psychological intervention takes more effect, and necessitating modification of the training procedure to allow for the effects of medication.

Clearly violence is a complex problem, and as such will often necessitate complex solutions. However, whilst violence as a whole may be complex, individual cases may be relatively simple and amenable to straightforward "technician" type approaches. Even such approaches however necessitate a minimal analysis of the problem: more complex problems require a detailed analysis and the development of individual solutions. Wherever possible treatment of problems of violence should be preceded by a detailed behavioural analysis which can then form the basis of subsequent intervention. Detailed assessment of the behaviour itself (its frequency, intensity etc.) permit not only evaluation of the analysis and consequent intervention, but also provide valuable information of use in revising such analyses. The armamentarium of procedures for dealing with violence is growing and their reported successes encouraging: it only remains to ensure that such procedures are used wisely and appropriately.

PRACTICAL IMPLICATIONS

The existence of a number of strategies for reducing violence implies the possibility of considerable improvement in the present state of affairs. Besides the development of a number of specific techniques applicable to problems of violence there exists also the possibility of detailed analyses leading to the design of specific interventions. Increasing knowledge regarding such interventions implies:

1. Traditional social and anthropological procedures have so far failed to make any substantial effect on the problem of violence. In particular judicial efforts towards suppression of violence by more and more severe measures have generally failed. Attempts at cultural change are in most cases either impractical, temporary or small scale with limited wider applicability.

2. Psychosurgery is becoming more and more difficult to justify as a strategy for dealing with violence, with many reports of failure and unwanted side effects. Similar problems are noted with attempts at hormonal manipulation, perhaps unsurprisingly given the difficulty of identifying their precise role in human aggression (see Chapter Three).

3. In the short term the use of drug treatments is effective in reducing violence, especially the use of powerful sedatives in emergencies. In the longer term however drugs may lose their effectiveness or produce undesirable side effects and their use here is more questionable. As outlined in Ch. 6 effective use of drug treatments may first require a detailed behavioural analysis of the problem.

4. Psychological procedures in widespread use can often be adapted to dealing with aggression. Such procedures may need to be used with caution however. Extinction, for example, may involve temporary rises in aggression, but, if this can be coped with, result in substantial reduction or elimination of the problem.

5. In addition to extinction such procedures as punishment and time out (TO) may be used. Most methods of punishment run the risk of eliciting reactive aggression, however, and may increase

rather than reduce the problem. TO involves the problem of determining a suitable duration, evidence suggesting that such periods should be kept as brief as possible, rarely exceeding two or three minutes.

6. Where the cooperation of the aggressor can be obtained a number of procedures may be considered. These include desensitisation to eliciting stimuli, Rational Emotive Therapy, assertiveness training and social skills training. Such procedures may often be combined into "anger control" packages.

7. In addition to the use of specific techniques the professional will often be able to provide a detailed analysis of a problem permitting a "tailor made" solution. Such an approach involves study of Antecedents, Behaviour and Consequences (the "ABC" paradigm) with attempts at Amelioration, Elimination and Compensation directed towards relevant factors.

8. Since it is not always possible to prevent aggressive incidents, professionals should be trained in their appropriate handling. The variety of forms that such aggression can take make rigid guidelines impossible. However general guidelines may be derived from what is known about violent processes, aimed at minimising those factors which increase the chances of aggression and maximising those which reduce the chances. Such measures include maintaining a minimal reaction to aggressive acts, in order to avoid reinforcement of operant aggression or the eliciting of reactive aggression. In addition actions should be such as to indicate that aggression is unlikely to succeed, including avoiding turning one's back on an aggressor, avoiding putting oneself in a vulnerable position etc. Finally actions should be aimed at producing behaviour incompatible with aggression, such as sitting down and relaxing.

9. The need to deal with an aggressive incident should always be seen as an indication of failure of prevention, and associated with subsequent enquiry about what can be learned from the incident for the future, and what steps need to be taken to help both aggressor and target.

10. Because of the complexity of violence, the chances of obtaining a satisfactory solution increase the more one has relevant information; in an ideal situation therefore considerable effort

will be addressed to the gathering of information and the analysis of the processes involved. In practice however it will often be necessary to take action on the basis of limited information. In either case it is important that data gathering procedures be as efficient as possible.

Chapter Eight

OBTAINING INFORMATION

It will be apparent from Chapter Seven that in order
to use even the simplest of techniques in treating
aggression some gathering of information is
necessary. If a detailed formulation of a problem
is to be made, the need for information is
correspondingly greater. In gathering information,
however, the first priority is to decide what kinds
of information are relevant. Obviously there is a
potential infinity of information about any
incident, most of which will bear little if any
relationship to the design of an intervention
strategy. It is important therefore to have, as far
as possible, a thorough understanding of the
processes of violence, in order to know what factors
are or are not likely to be relevant. It is for
this reason that so much space in the present work
has been devoted to theoretical issues.
    The ABC ("Antecedents-Behaviour-Consequences")
framework referred to in Chapter Seven provides a
convenient division of the factors which need to be
considered in investigating violence related
problems. Not only is it desirable to gather as
much relevant information as possible: in many
cases it will be essential to do so. Failure to
take account of all relevant factors may leave an
intervention doomed to failure. Each of the three
areas raises its own issues, however, and although
in practice all would need to be investigated, for
the present it is convenient to consider them
separately.

ANTECEDENTS

By "antecedents" is meant any event which, preceding
the violent episode, is in some way responsible for

its occurrence. In considering possible antecedents a number of issues need to be considered. It is important, in particular, to remember that an antecedent may actually precede a violent outburst by some considerable amount of time. In Patrick's (1967) study of a Glasgow gang (see Chapter Four) it was noted that an attack may have been precipitated by some earlier event. Thus the reason given for attacking one young woman had been that she had laughed at a gang member some time previously. An explanation of the attack woulld be inadequate if it failed to take note of this. Equally however a complete explanation would have to take into account other factors, in order to show not only why the attack occurred but why it occurred at that particular time. Some such factors would of course be trivial: the woman could not, for example, be attacked until she was present. Other factors however would also be relevant, including the presence of other gang members, the absence of authority figures etc. A search for relevant antecedents, then, needs to consider both the immediate and the distant precursors of an attack.

A second point to note is that, whilst some antecedents may be discrete events (e.g. an insulting remark, a threatening gesture etc.) others may be more diffuse. That is to say certain combinations of circumstance may constitute setting conditions for a violent episode. Such conditions may include such things as being in a particular place, in the company of certain individuals etc. Such factors would not in themselves produce violence, but may set the occasion for violence to be likely. Of particular note here are such factors as alcohol, not producing of violence in itself but setting the occasion for violence to occur.

Implicit in this is the notion that antecedents may interact in complex ways. At a basic level we may look for antecedents under the two headings of those aversive events which produce reactive aggression and those which act as discriminative stimuli for operant aggression. The fact that such antecedents may interact with each other however adds considerable complexity. Antecedents may act in combination with each other such that the effect of two together will be greater than the effect of one alone. Thus the occurrence of an insult from a rival gang member may have its impact greatly increased by the presence of a peer group before whom it is necessary to save face. The specific antecedent of the insult in conjunction with the presence of a peer group interact to increase the probability of a violent episode.

Antecedents may also have competing effects, such that one may serve to increase the probability of aggression whilst another serves to decrease it. Under such circumstances the final probability of an aggressive episode may be somewhere between the probabilities implied by any one of them alone. A friendly voice may reduce the probability of aggression, an insult increase it: the probability of aggression in response to a friendly-sounding insult may be somewhere in between. Finally it is important to remember that a combination of antecedents with individually similar effects need not produce a resultant effect in the same direction. Any one individual being offensive may elicit an aggressive response, but five such individuals together, far from being five times as likely to produce aggression, is more likely to produce escape.

Thus in looking for important antecedents it is necessary to search for events which may elicit reactive aggression and which may be discriminative for operant aggression. The effects of such antecedents may be masked, particularly by being separated in time from the event and by interacting with other, also relevant, antecedents. Such masking may be less of a problem where violence occurs repeatedly, enabling frequent "samples" of the violence to be taken and common features identified. Clarification may also sometimes be obtained by observing significant antecedents of non-violence: by identifying circumstances under which violence does not occur it is often possible to identify more easily those circumstances under which it does.

BEHAVIOUR

In any attempt to produce a treatment programme for problems of violence it is essential to gather information about the behaviour itself. At the very least it is valuable to gather information regarding the frequency of occurrence of the behaviour. Since one of the objectives of the intervention will be to eliminate the behaviour, or at least to reduce its frequency, careful assessment of the original rate of the behaviour will enable early detection of the effects of treatment. If information has not been precisely collected, it may be difficult to judge whether the rate of a behaviour is remaining the same, increasing slightly or decreasing slightly.

For this reason it has become the accepted practice in many treatment programmes to defer intervention until detailed information is available regarding the "normal" rate at which the individual is violent. Such estimates are then used as a baseline against which to assess the effects of intervention and hence are known as "baseline measurements". In many types of psychological intervention the therapist is exhorted to defer intervention until a stable baseline estimate is obtained. Obviously this will often be impossible in dealing with problems of violence, since there may be an urgent need for intervention. Nevertheless as stable and reliable an estimate as possible should be made in order that the treatment may be adequately evaluated: failure to do so may in the long term make it difficult if not impossible to determine which aspects of a treatment are effective, which ineffective and which may even be counter-productive.

In addition to the frequency of the behaviour, other measures may be of importance in particular cases. In particular the intensity and duration of a behaviour may be of relevance. To be able to change aggressive behaviour from a savage physical attack to verbal abuse may constitute a major improvement even if such episodes occur at the same frequency as previously. In a similar way to be able to reduce the duration of a violent episode may constitute an improvement despite frequency remaining unchanged.

In some circumstances it may be appropriate to subdivide the behaviour into different types, both for assessment and evaluation (see Chapter Ten). With one of our patients, for example, it became useful to assess separately violent behaviour directed towards other people (primarily his wife) and violence towards inanimate objects (primarily the fittings in their flat). During the first stages of treatment violence towards people decreased whilst violence against objects increased: had we taken a simple measure of "number of violent episodes" the treatment would have appeared to have no effect at all, since the overall frequency of attacks remained roughly consistent.

Besides its value in providing information for the evaluation of treatment, examination of the behaviour may give clues as to the types of process and factors involved. Thus a violent attack which escalates steadily and which stops abruptly on the victim's becoming submissive may be much more likely to reflect operant aggression, reinforced perhaps by the control gained over the victim, than a single lashing out in an uncontrolled way as may happen in some cases of reactive aggression. Such distinctions must be made with caution however; to determine with confidence the type of aggression (reactive or operant) involved it is necessary to identify the factors of which it is a function. Topography alone gives nothing more than the first clues of what processes may be involved, and in many (if not most) instances the two processes will give rise to behaviours which are physically indistinguishable. The form of the behaviour may however give more definite clues to the role of additional factors: unsteadiness, lack of coordination and slurring of speech may indicate physical factors such as alcohol intoxication. Efficient, well directed and practised attacks make the involvement of an overcontrolled personality unlikely. Whilst it would be unwise to use the topography of the behaviour alone as a guide to such factors, it seems likely that behavioural characteristics will often provide a starting point for further investigation.

CONSEQUENCES

In considering the consequences of a behaviour two particular types of event will be of particular interest; reinforcers and punishers. To some extent working in opposition to each other, the former will function as maintainers of operant aggression. The latter will serve to suppress aggressive behaviour in the short term, although the permanence of the effect may be open to question.

Much of what has been said about antecedents applies also to consequences. Thus just as a significant antecedent may precede a behaviour by some considerable period of time, so may a reinforcer maintain a behaviour even though it occurs some time after the behaviour. Whilst the same applies to punishers, it should be remembered that in both cases evidence suggests that the effect of consequences is considerably weakened by their being separated in time from the behaviour. Immediate consequences seem to be especially powerful in their effect on behaviour, suggesting that detection of significant events immediately following an aggressive episode may be of importance

Again mirroring the role of antecedents it is evident that consequences may interact in various ways. Thus the reinforcing effect of a gang member winning a fight may be intensified by the encouraging comments and praise of other gang members. Consequences and antecedents may of course also interact with each other. Certain individuals or events may come to act as discriminative stimuli because of their differential association with reinforcement. The institutionalised patient who on being violent is always given a "good talking to" by a particular staff member will, if such a "talking to" is reinforcing, come to perceive that staff member as a discriminative stimulus indicating that reinforcement is available for violent behaviour. It is of course obvious that the converse may occur and that antecedents may affect consequences: the individual who is told that another person is responsible for some grievance is likely to find signs of suffering by that person increasingly reinforcing.

In dealing with both antecedents and consequences a number of points are important. Perhaps the most pertinent of these is that the function of particular antecedents and consequences may be quite idiosyncratic to individuals. Thus events which most people would consider to be punishers may function as reinforcers to certain people: a number of studies for example have pointed to reinforcing effects of so-called punitive action. In particular it seems to be the case that the individual who is ignored for most of the time may find any contact with others reinforcing, even if such contact involves being shouted at, hit or otherwise "punished". Even such procedures as Time Out should not be assumed to have a punishing effect until it is established that the situation from which the individual is being withdrawn is one which would normally involve reinforcement. One mentally handicapped patient showed no decrement in violence when placed in a TO room following attacks on an individual attempting to give some tests. Eventually it became apparent that escape from an unpleasant testing situation, even to a TO room, was serving to reinforce rather than punish the violence. With some individuals reinforcers may have an unpredictably powerful effect: for one violent psychotic patient, for example, it was never possible to find a more powerful reinforcer than a cup of tea.

SOURCES OF INFORMATION

In gathering information about problems of violence
it is possible to draw on a number of sources.
Information may be obtained by direct observation or
indirectly by enquiring of individuals concerned
with the problem. Each of these sources is subject
to various types of error: nevertheless it will
often be possible, by being aware of this, to make
at least some allowance for error.

Observational Methods

In some cases it may actually be possible to
directly observe instances of aggression; a day
room in a psychiatric hospital, for example, or a
playroom in a nursery, may provide a setting for a
considerable amount of verbal, and some physical
aggression. Where possible such direct observation
can provide valuable information about each element
of the ABC paradigm. A number of issues are
relevant however. For instance, it will rarely be
possible for a single investigator to continuously
observe and record behaviour. A nurse on duty, for
example, will only be able to observe during those
hours allocated to that particular unit, and then
only when other duties do not compete. Typically,
rather than continuously observing a behaviour some
kind of sampling procedure is used, whereby the
individual of interest is observed at certain times
of the day and inferences drawn from this sample
about the behaviour in general. Whilst commonly
used in behaviour modification programmes, such
procedures may be problematic when it comes to
dealing with problems of violence. Since most
violent individuals are violent relatively
infrequently, it follows that a sampling procedure
is unlikely to coincide with the rare occasion when
violence does occur. Such observational procedures
are therefore only of limited value unless the
behaviour occurs at a fairly high frequency and is
sufficiently mild to permit continued observation.
The use of such time sampling with low frequency
behaviours can lead to misleading estimates of the
incidence of the behaviour (see e.g. Powell,
Martindale and Kulp 1976). Extreme violence of
course is likely to be recorded whenever it occurs,
drawing attention unavoidably to itself; but much
mild aggression may not be noticed by those who are

not directly involved.

Where time sampling procedures are to be used it is important that the observer has a clear idea of what to look for, and that unequivocal criteria for the occurrence of relevant events be established. Thus "being in an aggressive mood" would be a vague thing to look for, and the decision as to whether or not the individual was in such a mood might vary according to differences in the basis for such judgements between observers, variations in mood of the observers themselves etc. "Speaking to another individual in a raised voice" would be less vague although there may be room for disagreement as to what constituted a raised voice. "Striking another individual" might be even more precise. Increasing the precision of observational criteria provides for much greater confidence in the information obtained. Experimental work typically involves the use of more than one independent observer, measures of agreement being calculated to show the degree to which the information is subject to the individual characteristics of particular observers. If both observers independently show a high degree of agreement, this suggests that the information closely reflects what actually happened rather than such things as fluctuation in the mood or attentiveness of the observer. A low degree of agreement suggests that what actually happened was responsible for only part of the results, a good deal of the data reflecting idiosyncracies of the observers.

In practice however direct observation will rarely be possible of violent episodes. Whilst staff on duty in an institution may observe most of the violence which occurs, they will often be engaged on other duties when the episode begins, preventing careful observation of the antecedents. By having to deal with the violence itself it may be more difficult to observe carefully the consequences. Much of the information we obtain about violent behaviour must therefore be obtained indirectly: such indirect sources involve their own particular types of error.

Indirect Sources of Information
(i) The Offender
In many circumstances it will be possible to obtain a considerable amount of information from the individual responsible for the aggressive behaviour. Such a situation is particularly likely to arise

where the individual is presenting with problems of "temper control" or "anger control". Here the individual may be motivated to change, and by implication more likely to give honest information, than an individual who is happy with a current pattern of behaviour.

The most common procedure for eliciting information in such circumstances is undoubtedly the clinical interview. Such interviews may be structured, unstructured or contain both structured and unstructured elements. Questions asked in interviews may be relatively open ended (e.g. "Tell me how the problem seems to you") or relatively closed (e.g. "Is your temper harder to control than it was six months ago?"). In the former the interviewee is given plenty of scope in answering: in the latter a simple "yes" or "no" may be all that is required. In interviewing clients, especially for the first time, a frequently used technique is to begin with relatively open-ended questions, in order to obtain a wide base of information, progressing to relatively closed questions to explore points of detail. An exception to such a procedure may involve opening the interview with a number of innocuous relatively closed questions: such questions make few demands on interviewees and may help to put them at ease.

In interviewing subjects it may often be helpful to ask not only for their version of what happened in some episode, but also why they thought it happened. Of course there is no reason to expect that the individual will necessarily produce a correct analysis of the process, since most individuals will have little knowledge of the relevant principles. Nevertheless most will have a partial analysis and this may prove a useful starting point for further exploration of the problem.

Often the interaction between therapist and client will be necessary not only for an understanding of the problem but also for the design of the treatment. In the systematic desensitisation procedure described in Chapter Seven, for example, the client provides a list of irritating situations in which anger control is problematic: in collaboration with the therapist these are then grouped around central themes and arranged in order of difficulty. For such treatment to be effective it is obviously necessary to obtain a high degree of cooperation from the client concerned.

Besides the use of the interview, relevant

information may also be obtained by the use of inventories, questionnaires etc. Much of the early work on overcontrolled and undercontrolled personality, for example, involved the use of the MMPI, a pencil and paper personality questionnaire. In working with young people a number of procedures have been developed for rapid identification of potential reinforcers (see e.g. Homme 1971, Tharp and Wetzel 1969). One such procedure consists of a number of incomplete sentences of the form "I will do almost anything to get ..." together with a rating scale in which the reinforcers specified are rated for potential effectiveness. A further source of information has been the life history: the individual may be asked either to describe, or commonly to write, an account of their life from the earliest time they can remember until the present moment. Such a procedure provides at least two benefits. Firstly it provides in convenient form similar information to that which would be provided in a conventional history-taking. Secondly analysis of the way in which information is phrased may give clues as to attitudes, values etc. For example one violent individual, in writing about his adolescence, wrote "Round this time I used to go out with a gang of mates. One of them I remember was really great - he'd take anybody on, it didn't matter how big they were...". Such a comment suggests that such "fearlessness" is of great importance to the individual and led to the exploration of the role of aggression, "standing up to people" and fearlessness in gaining not only respect from others but also in gaining self-respect.

Besides the use of widely standardised rating scales, inventories, questionnaires etc. it is of course not unusual for individual hospitals, units etc. to devise their own scales for use with their particular clientele. Whilst such scales can be of particular value, it is desirable to check as far as possible their psychometric properties (for a brief account of psychometric principles see Owens 1984). Failure to fully understand the properties of the scales can lead to over-dependence on the information obtained thereby. Where such information is not available the information should obviously be regarded with more caution.

(ii) Information from Others
Besides the offender it is of course possible to

obtain a considerable amount of information from others who are involved in violence. Such sources of information include friends and relatives of those involved in violence, those involved in dealing with a violent episode (e.g. police, hospital staff) and of course the victim of the violence. With such individuals the most common procedure is of course the interview. Exactly what information is sought in interview will of course depend greatly on the relationship of the interviewee to the offender. Relatives may be able to give considerable amounts of life history information: friends' information about recent concerns or changes in the individual. Those involved in the violent incident may often be able to give information about the behaviour itself. Whilst each of these sources is subject to some degree of error, there will also be much of value in the information obtained.

Whilst victims, in particular, may be able to give considerable information regarding an attack, especial care should be taken in their interviewing. Reactions to being the subject of a violent attack vary considerably. Such reactions may include expected reactions like fear to less obvious ones like guilt ("I suppose I must have done something to bring it on") and denial ("It's all in the past now and I don't see the need to talk about it. It was nothing, really"). Such reactions will need to be handled with care and tact.

(iii) Written Records

Besides the information available from the various people concerned with violence, much can often be gained from written records. Many aggressive individuals have a considerable documentation of their violence with records in hospitals, schools, prisons etc. Not all of these will necessarily be available, but such records as can be obtained will normally be of considerable value. Court depositions, for example, will often give precise information regarding a behaviour together with its immediate antecedents and consequences. Hospital or prison records will often contain information regarding the frequency of occurrence of violent outbursts. Such information can reduce considerably the duration of baseline periods in assessment by looking back into the past. Often such records will also contain detailed information regarding the individual's history, likes and dislikes and so on.

By scanning such records it is possible to obtain a considerable amount of information in a fairly short time. A word of caution is in order however: often records from various sources (schools, prisons and hospitals for example) will repeat the same piece of information. Such repetition need not necessarily imply that such information can therefore be relied upon. It may be that the information appeared in the first record and was then subsequently copied from that into subsequent records, or that the individual is merely consistent in repeating the same incorrect information on successive occasions.

SOURCES OF ERROR IN INFORMATION

A problem with all of the sources of information discussed above is that they are, in various ways, subject to distortion. Such distortion may be inadvertent or intentional. In some cases the possibilities of such distortion will be obvious. Thus a violent individual detained in an institution may distort the information given in the hope of securing an earlier release. Such distortion may involve not only the behaviour but also the antecedents and consequences. A violent attack may be described as less extreme than it really was, or the injuries caused may be described as having been inflicted accidentally, the intention having been much less aggressive. Antecedents may be distorted in order to shift perception of blame towards the victim, consequences may be described as having been particularly severe in order to elicit sympathy and so on.

Deliberate distortion may also occur when an individual is otherwise trying to be cooperative. Thus information of which the individual is ashamed may be suppressed in the hope that successful treatment will be able to proceed in any case. In such circumstances it is important that the person interviewed understands that the information asked for is all relevant to the problem and why.

The offender is not of course the only person who may intentionally distort information. A victim, for example, may have many reasons for distorting information. Fear that they may be suspected of having brought the attack upon themselves may lead to distortion of antecedents. In many cases questions of compensation, insurance etc. will provide monetary incentives to distort information in particular ways. Friends and relatives, too, may deliberately distort information, often in the hope of reducing blame attributed to the offender. Undiscovered incidents in the individual's past may not be mentioned, for fear that these will put a loved one in a bad light. Embarassment, too, may lead to distortion: a partner may find it difficult, for example, to talk of an individual's violence during sexual behaviour.

Written records may often be less susceptible to distortion, often being compiled by those who have no vested interest one way or another. However much of the information in records will have been obtained from the sources described above, and will therefore be subject to the same types of error. In addition some records will be subject to deliberate distortion. Court depositions, for example, will normally be challenged by opposing barristers: it is important that the only information included be that which can stand up as admissible evidence in a court of law. A well prepared statement therefore will usually omit reference to anything which is at all uncertain since to include it would run the risk of the statement later being discredited by a skilful lawyer.

Besides such intentional sources of distortion, other errors will inadvertently decrease the accuracy of information. In remembering, human beings tend to structure their recollections in such a way as to make sense, even when no such structure was apparent in the original incidents. Decades of research has shown that people will tend to "adjust" their memory if this makes more sense of the world. Other factors will affect both perception and recollection of incidents. Motivational factors, for instance will affect perceptual processes, especially when the material to be perceived is in any way doubtful or ambiguous. The individuals concerned will be quite unconscious of such distortions and sincerely believe the information they give.

Inadvertent distortion may also be introduced when people overestimate their own knowledge. Thus relatives or friends may feel they have such intimate knowledge of an offender that their having committed some offence is inconceivable to them. In "The Beast of Jersey", for example, the wife of a man convicted of thirteen sexual assaults on young children described how she never suspected her husband. His long night time strolls, the bonfires on which he was thought to have burned incriminating evidence, his refusal to participate in the mass

fingerprinting of island residents in the search for
the offender, all at the time had plausible
explanations. Only after his arrest and the
production of evidence in court did the significance
of much of his behaviour become apparent. Until
then she had been totally convinced of her husband's
innocence, being for example quite happy to leave
her own young children (his stepchildren) in his
care (Paisnel 1972).

The fact that information is rarely completely
reliable does not of course imply that it should be
ignored. Imperfect information is still better than
no information at all, especially when the user is
forewarned about possible inaccuracies. In addition
to such information however it will often be
necessary to devise specific recording procedures
for episodes of violence: such procedures may be of
particular importance in institutional settings.
The exact form of such records will of course depend
on the nature of the setting but a number of general
points may be made. Firstly the procedure should
adequately record significant features of the
antecedents, the behaviour and the consequences.
Secondly records should be kept of exactly who was
involved in both the incident itself and the
measures taken to deal with it. In addition the
person completing the record should be identified,
as should any additional factors which might
possibly be of relevance, such as medication,
alcohol ingestion etc. In preparing such procedures
it is common for "routine" information to be
recorded without any clear idea of why such
information might be included: this should be
guarded against, or records may become swamped with
irrelevant information. This implies a clear
purpose to a recording procedure, and from the
outset its role should be established. Thus if its
purpose is to gather information about violence and
psychiatric categorisation then a diagnosis may be
recorded: but if the purpose is to help in devising
an intervention programme for the individual's
violent behaviour such information is unlikely to be
of benefit since such diagnoses typically remain
constant through a treatment programme. By asking
exactly what difference the answers to a question
will actually make to treatment a number of items
can commonly be eliminated: the treatment will
often be independent of such information.
Information needs to be gathered only in as much as
it will affect a subsequent decision regarding
treatment.

It will be apparent, then, that a number of sources of information are available to the investigator. Whilst none is perfect, the use of several sources of information will sometimes provide a check on their reliability (though if each source is subject to the same type of error the check will of course be ineffective). In getting such information, however, the individual will rapidly become overwhelmed by a mass of data: it is necessary therefore to collate, condense and organise such information and use it to produce an understanding of the problem and to identify possible interventions.

PRACTICAL IMPLICATIONS

Since the causal factors are potentially quite complex, it is necessary to gather as much useful information as possible when attempting to solve problems of aggression. This implies the consideration of a number of issues relevant to the gathering of information including:

1. The Antecedents-Behaviour-Consequences ("ABC") framework provides a useful structure within which to organise data collection. Failure to gather information about all three is likely to result in an incomplete or distorted picture of the problem.

2. Each of the three may be complex and interact in subtle ways. Effects may be immediate and/or delayed with the effect of one factor being completely transformed depending on the presence or absence of another.

3. The various factors involved may have quite unusual roles to play in specific problems. For example a consequence which would punish most people's behaviour may serve to reinforce aggression in some individuals. The effect of different factors should therefore be assessed directly, not inferred or guessed at.

4. A number of sources of information may be available and it will often be useful to draw on several of these. Each has its own advantages and disadvantages however, and few if any will give a completely unbiased picture of the problem. Care must be taken not to place too much faith in any single source of information.

5. Even where the information available seems to be correct in itself it should be treated with caution, since certain information may have been omitted. A court deposition, for example, may contain only what is known with reasonable certainty and omit much potentially useful information about which there is slight doubt.

Chapter Nine

APPROACHES TO INTERVENTION

Having obtained information from as many sources as possible, it is then necessary to make use of this information in the selection or design of an intervention procedure. The amount of information required will depend to some extent upon the approach being taken to intervention. A simple technique-based approach may require only the identification of a few major factors: a problem-solving approach may require a much greater understanding of the ongoing processes and their aetiology. Either way it is necessary that the information obtained be organised and collated into a manageable form.

Making Sense of Information
An obvious first step in the classification of information is to divide the potentially important factors into antecedents, behaviours and consequences. Such a problem is relatively straightforward since such classification requires little more than a knowledge of chronological sequence. It must however be remembered that the humiliation of losing a fight, for example, may serve as a punisher of fighting but an antecedent of a later poisoning attempt. Moreover the behaviours may not have such obvious differences. Losing a fight may punish "fair" fighting but constitute a significant antecedent of a surprise attack: to the casual observer the behaviours may be indistinguishable despite the different causal role played by the losing of the fight.

A further step in the analysis of information involves identifying factors as relating to specific processes in aggression. Thus certain antecedents may have obvious aversive properties: these can be grouped as possible elicitors of reactive aggression. Depending on the consequences of the aggressive behaviour these may also constitute negative reinforcers for the behaviour. Thus the receipt of bad news may elicit reactive aggression: violence towards hospital staff who inform relatives of the death of a patient is not uncommon, for example, even though such aggression will have no effect on the bad news itself. Other aversive events may themselves be affected by aggressive behaviour however: the young mother who, helpless in the face of her baby's constant crying, flings the baby violently into a cot may do so as a reaction to the stress of the noise and her apparent helplessness. The consequent stunning and silencing of the child, however, whilst producing anxiety, fear and guilt may also have a reinforcing effect in removing the constant crying and giving at least a temporary illusion of control. In the latter case the same antecedent is implicated in both reactive and operant processes.

In identifying operant processes it is of course necessary to identify both significant antecedents and significant consequences. In general any consequence of violent behaviour should be examined for possible reinforcing effects. Even if the consequence is, overall, regarded as being unpleasant this does not preclude its having some reinforcing properties. To be struck by a person whom one has taunted and teased may not in itself be pleasant, but to the extent that it shows that the taunting has been successful, to be hit may have reinforcing properties.

In considering operant aggression it is of course also important to consider the role of antecedents as discriminative stimuli. Discriminative stimuli may be of one of two kinds: those that indicate the unavailability of reinforcement, and hence reduce the probability of operant aggression, and those which indicate the availability of reinforcement and hence increase the probability of operant aggression.

An example of the former might be the presence of some individual or group of individuals who would prevent aggression occurring and hence leave attempts at violence unreinforced. The presence of a large police contingent near a street gang, or of a parent near an aggressive child may be sufficient to make it clear that aggressive behaviour is unlikely to be reinforced. Other discriminative stimuli may make the probability of aggressive behaviour high by virtue of their indicating a high likelihood of reinforcement. Outward signs of wealth such as fine clothes, expensive jewellery etc. may indicate to a potential attacker that the potential for financial gain resulting from an attack is relatively high. Such stimuli would, for that individual in those circumstances, constitute positive discriminative stimuli. It should be noted that such discriminative stimuli may function by indicating that reinforcement is more likely or that the reinforcement is more substantial, or both. Thus the wearing of a badge saying "British Karate Association" may indicate that reinforcement is less likely but may still serve a positive function by indicating that the status resulting from a successful encounter will be that much higher. The identification of the particular function of a stimulus is not therefore predictable in any simply way but requires a detailed knowledge of its relationship to reinforcement contingencies.

Not all factors will of course relate directly to operant or reactive aggression but may rather function as modifiers of those factors which do relate directly. Thus drugs and alcohol, for example, do not in themselves produce aggression but may play a part in modifying the effects of other factors which do. The role of such contributory factors should not of course be neglected, since these may be of crucial importance in analysing and dealing with problems. Neglect of the role of drugs reducing reactive aggression, for example, may lead to the mistaken assumption that such aggression plays no significant part in a problem, only to find that such aggression once again becomes a problem when the drug is no longer available.

Having (at least provisionally) identified the role of the various factors thought to be involved it is then necessary to map out the relationships between them. Some of the factors will interrelate in simple ways, others may be complex. As noted in Chapter Seven it is not unusual for the interrelationships to involve some form of feedback, as when aggression leads to reinforcement and so on. Such a "vicious circle" will have the effect of stabilising the aggression at some maximum level (either the maximum rate at which aggression can occur or the maximum rate at which reinforcement can occur).

It may also be desirable at this stage to distinguish historical factors which no longer apply, but which are of significance in understanding the development of the behaviour, and current factors, still operating and serving to maintain the behaviour. Thus an individual may have taken boxing lessons as a child: as an aggressive adult the boxing lessons may no longer be relevant to the maintenance of the aggressive behaviour but may nevertheless be important in understanding how the aggressive patterns of behaviour evolved in the first place. Historical factors may be of significance for a number of reasons. Although a factor which is no longer operating is rarely likely to be of direct significance in the maintenance of behaviour, such a factor will often have a long-term indirect effect by creating a situation which does continue. Thus having taken boxing lessons as a child is unlikely to be of direct relevance to adult behaviour, such lessons having perhaps stopped some 20 or 30 years earlier; there may however be an indirect relevance in that the acquired skills, remaining long after the lessons cease, influence such things as the probability that operant aggression will be successful. Noting the factors which appear to have been of importance in the development of the behaviour may give useful clues to those involved in its maintenance.

Historical factors may also be important when it comes to predicting the outcome of any intervention. In particular if the circumstances which originally lld to the development of the aggression are likely to recur it is necessary to not only gain control of the aggressive behaviour but also to prepare the client for future encounters with the original set of circustances: failure to do so may result in the individual re-learning the aggressive behaviour as was done originally.

It is possible then to identify a number of discrete stages in the analysis of data relevant to problems of violence. These may be summarised as follows:

(a) Listing of all factors, events, stimuli, people etc. which may be of relevance to the problems. In the early stages it may be appropriate to include in such a list any feature which seems in any way unusual or idiosyncratic, even if not having any immediately obvious relevance to the violent behaviour.

(b) Dividing up of the features listed into those which are historical and those which are current, those which are antecedents and those which are consequences, those which seem relevant to operant and those which seem relevant to reactive

aggression and so on. Such a division will usually
result in a number of factors falling into more than
one category (e.g. being involved in both operant
and reactive aggression, or being of both historical
and current interest). At this stage a number of
factors will not be easily classifiable, that is to
say their role in the aggression may not be clear.
Such a difficulty may reflect a true irrelevance of
such factors or simply that more information about
them is still needed.

(c) Grouping of similar factors under a common
heading. Often it will be possible to identify
groups of factors which are similar in their
relationship to the problem. Thus "being joked
about by friends", "being ignored by a shop
assistant", and "being spoken to patronisingly" may
for one individual all be examples of "not being
treated with respect". Clustering factors in this
way can lead to a substantial reduction in the
amount of data the investigator has to handle: it
is important however to keep open the possibility
that not all the factors included under one heading
may actually belong there and to be ready to
reclassify as necessary.

(d) Mapping out of interrelationships between
factors or clusters of factors. Identifying such
interrelationships can often be made easier by
noting the factors/clusters on paper and connecting
with lines those which affect each other. The
resulting network will then reveal such processes as
feedback loops of importance in intervention.

Such a mapped out set of interrelationships
constitutes a preliminary formulation of the
problem. By examining such a formulation it should
be possible to see how the behaviour "makes sense"
in terms of the factors of which it is a function.
Where the behaviour does not "make sense" is a sign
of where further information is needed. If such
information can be obtained the formulation can be
further refined. If not, it may be necessary to
proceed on the basis of what information is
available. Either way the existence of such a
formulation, even if only tentative, provides a
basis for the selection of an intervention
procedure.

POINTS OF INTERVENTION

Having obtained an understanding of the violent
behaviour it then becomes necessary to decide upon

an appropriate plan of intervention. In deciding what action to take, various issues need to be considered. Any intervention will operate by either bringing about a change in the relevant variables, the relationships between them, or both. Thus the variables may be changed by such procedures as extinction, such that the reinforcers which originally followed the behaviour no longer do so. Alternatively the events themselves may remain, action being taken to change the type of relationship the events have with the behaviour. Thus it may not be possible to stop one individual being confronted with another who is disliked even when such meetings result in violence. If the two can become friendly, however, their meetings may continue but no longer result in violence. The events still physically occur, but they no longer have the same functional significance.

Where the intervention is to be based on a series of techniques such as assertion training, desensitisation, self-control etc. the information required may, in the first instance consist merely of noting whether the process involved is primarily operant or reactive. Where it is desired to produce a "customised" intervention however it will be necessary to examine all of the relevant factors and decide which will constitute the prime targets for an intervention programme. Reference has already been made to the potential importance of feedback loops and where these are found they will normally constitute a prime target for intervention. Failure to do so leaves open the possibility that whatever procedure is adopted its effects will last only until the feedback loop begins to operate again, after which the behaviour will once again increase to a maximum.

Other factors will of course also need to be taken into account in choosing points for intervention. Whether or not it is possible to gain access to relevant variables will often determine a strategy - where aggression is reinforced by the observation of the victim's suffering or injury, interference with reinforcement may be imposible: a victim cannot simply decide not to suffer or bruise. In planning intervention it will usually also be desirable to consider not simply the present environment but also future environments: it is of little value eliminating an individual's violence by simply imposing constant supervision if it is eventually hoped to return such an individual to an unsupervised setting. This is not of course to say that artificial procedures need never be used, simply that a transition from the artificiality of the programme to the processes of the normal environment should be programmed. Thus lavish praise may be used in teaching social interaction: once the skills have been learned, however, such artificial reinforcement needs to be gradually faded out, the natural reinforcers of day-to-day living serving to maintain the behaviour.

EXAMPLES

The preparation of interventions may be illustrated by taking a couple of examples from clinical practice. Inevitably the accounts to be given are much oversimplified: they do however give a rough guide as to how such procedures might be applied.

Case 1. Jack

Jack was referred by his General Practitioner, also a friend of the family, following a long history of angry and aggressive outbursts. The 20 year old son of a wealthy businessman, he lived a somewhat reckless life, running up debts, gambling and drinking, neglecting his work in his father's business. His father would typically "bail out" Jack when he got into difficulties but any attempt to improve control by the father was met with a violent outburst. Eventually this built up to crisis point.

Investigation took the form of interviews with the son and father from which a number of questions emerged including (a) did the aggression constitute reactive aggression, in anger at his father, operant aggression, reinforced by his father's acquiescence, or both? (b) If the father's behaviour was indeed reinforcing the aggression, why did the father continue to employ Jack and to bail him out of his difficulties?

The answers to these questions were in detail too complex for consideration here. Briefly, however, it became apparent that Jack had a long history of achieving his aims through violence such as fights at school and at home. As he grew up, however, this inevitably became a matter of more serious concern. His parents, it appeared, had neglected Jack in his childhood: a chronically sick brother had taken a good deal of time, in addition to which his father had been busy building up the family business. By the time the brother died Jack had, with little parental control, already developed a number of aggressive patterns of behaviour. Increasing realisation of the way in which Jack had been neglected, however, had left the father with strong guilt feelings, leaving him desperate to make things up to him and reluctant to refuse his wants. Jack soon learned that he could play on this and obtain whatever he wanted from his father. In this way he obtained an executive position in the business, a fast car and an expense account. By the time he had crashed two cars and run up a number of overdrafts the father realised that he could no longer maintain Jack's lifestyle. Attempts to clamp down on Jack's lifestyle led to threats and violence and eventually to the referral.

Clearly what had happened was that Jack had in early life learned that aggression could be used to obtain power, status and material benefit without the constraints of parental supervision. Later he found that he could pressurise his father into giving him considerable support, laying the foundations of operant aggression. When his father later began to refuse, the effect was that of introducing extinction: the aversiveness of finding that previously successful behaviour was no longer being reinforced led to an outbreak of reactive aggression. This led his father into compromising and negotiating, thus reinforcing the new (higher) level of aggression. Needless to say the same thing happened with the next refusal, the violence escalated further and so on. The violence thus consisted of a mixture of operant aggression reinforced by the power gained over his father and reactive aggression in response to his father's (half-hearted) attempts at extinction. Such an analysis implied two main lines of attack on the problem. Of obvious importance was the breakup of the reinforcement contingency (being prepared for another outbreak of violence but this time with a determination to avoid reinforcement) in conjunction with reinforcement of more positive behaviour (attending for therapy, working efficiently in the business etc.). Secondly family therapy was suggested as a means of modifying the relationship between Jack and his father and to help deal with father's long standing feelings of guilt towards Jack.

Case 2. Susan
From quite a different point on the social scale came Susan, in her early twenties and living on a

council estate. Totally failing to calm her baby,
Susan had missed many nights sleep and finally, in a
moment of despair, thrown him away from her,
fracturing his leg and skull. The baby was taken
into care and Susan referred in the hope that she
might at some point be able to take the baby back.
Important questions included (a) why had Susan not
sought help from family, friends or official
agencies before reaching the end of her tether and
(b) what was the likelihood of her reacting
similarly if the same circumstances recurred?

Information here was gathered from a number of
sources including Susan, her husband, the social
worker responsible, the foster mother and official
records. The incident itself seemed to be a
straightforward example of reactive aggression in
response to the continued crying and exacerbated by
the sleepless nights. Susan's failure to obtain
help from other sources was however more of a
problem. Closer examination of Susan's history
revealed a number of important features. Most of
her adolescence had been spent in care: pregnant at
14, she had been given an abortion and placed in a
children's home. This had produced several effects
including a mistrust of her mother, who was
perceived as having thrown her out when in need, and
a considerable amount of guilt. These events seemed
also to have left her with a very low opinion of
herself. In addition her husband was violent
towards her, her father in prison on a theft charge.
The foster mother reported that the baby was indeed
a difficult child but was becoming less so as he
grew older. Susan herself presented as an
unassertive, possibly overcontrolled, individual.

Analysis of these and a number of other factors
suggested that Susan's lack of assertiveness was a
function of her guilt regarding both her adolescent
pregnancy and the subsequent abortion which she felt
she had been "pushed into having". This in addition
to her poor self-image had left her feeling
unentitled to assert herself: by not attempting to
assert herself she never learned to do so, making
her feel even more inadequate and setting up a
feedback loop. Her relationships with husband and
family were so poor that she was unable to turn to
them for help.

Therapy, then, aimed at such issues as relieving
guilt and encouraging greater assertiveness. A
Rational-Emotive framework enabled her to, for
example, compare the way she blamed herself with her
unwillingness to blame another fourteen year old in

the same position. Increased assertiveness followed, she instituted divorce proceedings and built up a new social network including the foster mother. Eventually the baby was returned to her, the foster mother remaining as a resource to whom Susan could turn if things became too difficult.

In this case then the reactive aggression was dealt with directly by removing the main eliciting factor (the difficult baby). In order to insure against a recurrence of the incident however alternative responses were built up whereby Susan would feel able to assert herself and make demands on other people like the foster mother. It is not possible to say whether or not this assertiveness was also a factor in her seeking a divorce, but such a step in any case served to reduce the chronic stress under which she normally existed.

Case 3. Peter

Peter was a student at a large university. Normally a pleasant and friendly person, he was characterised by outbursts towards his fellow students when he had been out drinking. His peers became concerned, and eventually he contacted the student counsellor who referred him to a clinical psychologist. Whilst it was clear that his violence was a function of alcohol intake, other factors also needed to be identified in order to determine why alcohol should have such and effect.

On interviewing Peter, it became clear that he felt himself to be something of an outsider at university. Coming from a rather tough, working-class background he saw the largely middle-class society of university as threatening and difficult. Himself he saw as inadequate and socially clumsy amongst his sophisticated peer group.

Before coming to university Peter had been a member of a street gang where fighting had been commonplace and a sign of masculinity, giving increased status. Once at university such behaviour was no longer appropriate.

What appeared to be happening was that violent behaviour had in the past been reinforced. On coming to university however this no longer constituted a method of "proving" himself, something which his self-perception of awkwardness necessitated him doing. His drinking appeared to be a function both of his distress at not fitting in and his attempt to demonstrate his masculinity by showing an impressive alcohol capacity. This meant that the self control by which he normally controlled his aggression became impaired and that he returned to his old, violent methods of attempting to gain acceptance.

Treatment in this case, then, was directed at building up Peter's confidence within his social group and teaching him non-violent ways of gaining acceptance. Challenging of his irrational beliefs regarding appropriate routes to social acceptance and building on his other strengths enabled him to learn to fit into university life without the use of violence.

Obviously it is not possible in a few short case histories to do anything more than illustrate how problems might be approached. It has been necessary to omit many of the relevant details, only the major features of each case being included. The cases themselves, however, are in no way atypical: the same kinds of process will be familiar to anyone working in the field of violence. Yet the cases are also each unique in their particular composition reflecting the variety of problems coming under the heading of violence. In both cases, however, and many more besides, it is possible to see the application of a particular strategy: that of gathering information, formulating the problem, and on the basis of the formulation designing an intervention.

PRACTICAL IMPLICATIONS

The steps from gathering information to intervening
are not necessarily straightforward. A number of
stages need to be passed through, each with its own
important aspects. Amongst these are:

1. In order to make use of information it is
necessary that it be reduced to a manageable level.
A convenient basis for classification is in terms of
antecedents, behaviour and consequences, though such
a distinction will sometimes be rather arbitrary.

2. A second aspect of classification is in terms of
the basic processes involved. Some of the factors
will relate to operant processes, some to reactive
processes, and some to both.

3. The functions of certain factors may be quite
complex, serving perhaps to enhance one form of
aggression whilst inhibiting another. Similarly the
function of one variable may be affected by the
presence or absence of others.

4. Mapping out of the various factors involved in
terms of their relationship to the behaviour will
enable a "model" of the aggression to be developed
in terms of which the problem may be understood.
Such a model will often involve a number of feedback
loops serving to stabilise the problem in one way or
another.

5. Identification of the functions of the behaviour
provides a basis both for understanding the
behaviour and for developing an intervention. Often
the analysis will suggest that action may be taken
to deal with some other problem whose link with the
aggression may not be immediately obvious. To the
extent that the violence resulted from such a
problem a successful elimination will also deal with
the consequential violence.

Chapter Ten

EVALUATION OF INFORMATION

Having analysed a problem and designed and implemented a possible solution, it remains only to consider procedures designed to assess the results. The evaluation of intervention procedures involves two related but distinct issues. In the first place it is necessary to assess whether or not there actually has been any change in the problem behaviour. A successful intervention is likely to reduce either the frequency or the intensity of violence (or both). Secondly it may be important not only to determine whether any change has taken place but also to decide whether the change can reasonably be attributed to the intervention rather than to other factors. How, and the extent to which this is done, will depend upon the specific factors in each situation including the purposes for which the information is required. In particular it may be necessary to evaluate intervention with respect to the behaviour of individuals, of groups of individuals or with respect to changes in the amount of violence observed in particular settings.

Evaluation with Individuals
Obviously in determining whether or not the amount of violence shown by an individual has been reduced it is necessary first to have good information regarding the pre-treatment or "baseline" rate of the behaviour. At its simplest level evaluation may consist of nothing more than continuing to monitor the behaviour during and after intervention and noting whether the amount of violence is indeed lower following treatment. By plotting a graph of the level of behaviour it is possible to make an immediate visual comparison of the level of the violence during and after treatment comparing this

with the baseline level. In this way it is possible
to decide not only whether or not the problem has
been reduced, but also to determine whether or not
the reduction is more than could be accounted for by
simple day-to-day variation in the behaviour. Such
evaluation consists of two clear phases - before the
intervention started and after the intervention
started. Labelling these as A and B, the procedure
as a whole has come to be known as an AB design.

Whilst such a procedure is often adequate for
the determination of whether behaviour has in fact
changed, however, it still leaves open the question
of whether the change can reasonably be attributed
to the intervention procedure. Obviously at the
time an intervention begins a number of other
changes may have occurred which are themselves
coincidentally responsible for the reduction in the
behaviour. For example it may be that on the same
day a treatment programme is begun the individual
who elicits most of the aggression from the subject
moves away, or that the media begin a campaign
against violence, or that the subject falls ill and
so on. Any of these could actually be responsible
for the reduction in the problem and result in the
effectiveness of the treatment programme being
overestimated.

In many approaches to changing problem behaviour
an attempt has been made to identify more precisely
the role of the intervention by later reversing the
procedure. Thus in an attempt to eliminate a
problem behaviour using an extinction procedure four
distinct phases may be identified: an initial
baseline phase when pre-treatment data is collected,
an extinction phase during which an attempt is made
to avoid reinforcing the behaviour, and then a third
phase during which a return is made to baseline
conditions. In this "second baseline" phase the
supposed reinforcer is once again made available
contingent upon the problem behaviour. If the
supposed reinforcer was indeed responsible for the
behaviour in the first place, the problem should
return to its original level. Following this it is
then possible to return once again to the extinction
phase and produce a final elimination of the
behaviour.

Such an approach, known for obvious reasons as
an ABAB design, provides much greater confidence
that the changes in behaviour are indeed a result of
the changed conditions in each phase, since for
other factors coincidentally to change in step with
the treatment programme is unlikely. In practice

however such procedures will often be either impractical or undesirable. It is difficult, for example, to reverse the effect of teaching someone to relax in the presence of previously irritating stimuli. Even if it were possible to do so it is unlikely that a return, even if temporary, of the violent behaviour would be seen as acceptable. This often means that the evaluation of individual programmes is restricted to determining whether a change has occurred, leaving open the question of whether the change might reasonably be attributed to the programme rather than external factors.

An alternative approach to evaluation is provided by the so-called "multiple baseline" technique. Here the behaviour to be changed is dealt with in a piecemeal fashion, intervention being applied successively to different aspects of the behaviour (or to totally different behaviours where several are to be changed). Thus in a psychiatric hospital a time-out programme (see Chapter Seven) may be introduced in the first instance only to deal with an individual's aggression towards others in a particular setting such as a day room. Initial baseline data is however collected over a wide range of behaviours (e.g. aggression towards property, aggression in the dining room etc.). Since the intervention is specific to one particular part of the behaviour it is to be expected that only this part of the behaviour will show substantial changes: the remaining aspects of the behaviour, not being subject to the TO contingency, should remain largely unaffected. At a later stage the TO contingency can be extended to other types of behaviour, settings etc. To the extent that changes in the behaviours reflect the successive application of the TO to the various aspects, increased confidence can be gained that the changes are indeed a result of the programme.

A number of other procedures exist for the evaluation of experimental manipulations with individuals or with small numbers of subjects. (See e.g. Sidman, 1960, Hersen and Barlow 1971.) Often however evaluation of a procedure will extend beyond its application to a single individual to the assessment of treatment of several people, either considered as a single group, a number of sub-groups or a number of repetitions of individual studies.

Evaluation with a Number of Individuals.

At a very simple level the evaluation of treatment programmes with several people may consist of nothing more than a number of repetitions of the procedures used with individuals. Often however the availability of information on a number of people will extend the number of potential approaches to evaluation. The multiple baseline approach, for example, can be modified such that instead of taking baseline data on a number of behaviours on a single individual the baselines are instead taken on a single behaviour in a number of individuals. The frequency of violent outbursts by delinquent adolescents in a community home, for example, may be monitored for a number of problem individuals. If an intervention is then introduced at different times for each individual it should be possible to demonstrate that each individual's behaviour shows substantial changes only following the introduction of the treatment programme for that individual.

Often, particularly in large-scale research studies, the behaviour of the group, expressed as some kind of average, will be considered in preference to the behaviour of individuals. Thus the average frequency of aggressive incidents in a group may be considered before and after implementation of treatment. Such a procedure is akin to the AB design with an individual, except that here the measure of interest is the average behaviour of the group members rather than the behaviour of any one member. As with the individual AB design the risk remains that any change noted is actually due to some coincident external factor.

Typically where the average effect of a treatment on a group of individuals constitutes an acceptable measure, some kind of statistical approach to evaluation will be considered. A basic design here might involve dividing a group of potential subjects in advance into two subgroups: one of the groups (the "experimental" or "treatment" group) then receives treatment, whilst the remaining group (the "control" group) is exposed to exactly the same conditions (measures etc.) but not actually treated. Since the two groups are identical but for the way in which they have been treated, any subsequent difference, it is argued, must reflect the effects of treatment. Numerous extensions to this basic design have been developed permitting the investigation not only of effects of treatments, but also the interactions of such effects with factors such as subject characteristics, types of problem behaviour and so on. Such designs are too complex for consideration here, but are widely documented in texts on research methods (see e.g. Kerlinger, 1972).

Evaluation with Settings

It is worth noting that besides attempting to reduce the amount of violence associated with certain people, it will sometimes be necessary to reduce the amount of violence associated with certain settings. Often some particular parts of an organisation or institution will be associated with an unduly high level of violence: in hospitals, for example, Accident and Emergency Units (Casualty departments) may be the scene for a much higher level of violence than remaining sections of the hospital. Reduction of violence cannot be accomplished by dealing with the aggressors, since these will usually be different on each occasion. On the other hand an assessment and formulation of the problem might suggest a number of strategies which would reduce the problem, such as changing the seating arrangements, training staff to recognise and calm potentially violent patients etc. Here the success or otherwise of the action taken can be assessed in a similar way to the assessment of individual change, but taking such measures as the frequency of violent episodes within the unit, the severity of such episodes (as measured by such factors as the severity of damage done or injury caused). Figures of this kind can then be analysed in the same way that figures for individual people are evaluated, the success or otherwise of the programme being identified accordingly.

Problems of Evaluation

Although the principles of evaluation are relatively simple, in practice a number of problems will need to be considered. The information on which the evaluation is based, for example, will be less than perfect, with a number of factors causing some degree of bias and distortion (as discussed in Chapter Eight). Various decisions need to be made with respect to both the choice of data and the strategy adopted for its use. Whereas often it will be possible to measure directly changes in the amount of violence, on many occasions this will not be possible and indirect assessments may have to be taken. Such measures may include diaries kept by individuals in treatment, reports obtained during interview, self-ratings by aggressors of experienced hostility and so forth. In considering evaluation with groups of individuals additional similar problems may occur. Whether or not to compare post-treatment aggressiveness between experimental or control groups, or relative changes in aggressiveness between the groups, may affect the appearance of the results. In addition the consideration of group results may also raise less obvious issues in the choice of measure: a treatment may for example not change the average hostility of a group yet have substantial effects on some of the group members. It may be, for example, that of a group many of the members were improved slightly by a treatment but one was made substantially worse: the overall average may be little different to pre-treatment, but it would be a mistake to conclude that the treatment had no effect.

In addition the evaluation of some treatment programme will usually wish to consider the extent to which results obtained are maintained over a period of time. The identification of an appropriate time period will often depend on the nature of the intervention: a Time Out programme for example may not be expected to continue once the Time Out contingency is allowed to lapse: the teaching of general self-control skills however might be expected to continue indefinitely. Even this latter however may be subject to some distortion at follow-up. The person concerned may, for example, have retained the ability to exert self-control but may now be in a situation where it is no longer appropriate to do so.

In general the answers to such problems will not be decided on a general basis: rather the best answer in each situation will depend on specific characteristics of that situation. The analysis and formulation of the problem will thus be of crucial importance in determining the kind of evaluation. If the formulation involves the individual being motivated to change, for example, a different credence may be given to self reports of improvement than if the formulation involves only external pressures to appear changed (e.g. in a prisoner due for parole consideration). Thus with evaluation as well as intervention the formulation of the problem will often provide guidelines regarding the best course of action.

Influence of Evaluation on Formulation

As a final note it is important to remember that, besides the formulation directing the evaluation, the evaluation will also affect the formulation. Typically the information available regarding a problem will permit several alternative formulations, with there often being insufficient evidence to choose between them. Under such circumstances a decision may be taken to go ahead with an intervention based on one of the possible models, perhaps the one which is most plausible, or the one which implies greatest potential for intervention.

If clearly understood, such a formulation will imply quite definite consequences for any intervention programme. If aggressive behaviour is believed to be under the control of a particular reinforcer, for example, such a formulation of the problem will clearly imply a reduction in the frequency of the behaviour (perhaps after an initial extinction-induced increase) when the reinforcement contingency is eliminated. If a programme designed to eliminate such a contingency fails to reduce the violence then the formulation obviously needs to be revised. That is to say, the failure of the intervention provides further information, thus permitting refinement of the formulation or rejection of that formulation in favour of an alternative.

It should, incidentally, be noted that a further possibility exists, to the effect that the formulation of the problem may be correct but that the intervention has failed to control the relevant factors. Thus if it is believed that a psychiatric patient's violence is reinforced by attention from ward staff, an intervention may fail not because the analysis was incorrect but simply because the attempt at intervention (withdrawing attention from the violence, and transfering it to some more positive behaviour) was not carried out: the staff concerned may, for example, not have understood what was required, or may have disagreed with the programme or failed to carry out the programme for other reasons. In evaluating a treatment procedure, therefore, it will often be necessary to check that the procedures were actually carried out before rejecting the formulation on which they were based. Evaluation will therefore normally involve both

156

evaluation of the treatment programme and of its effects on the violent behaviour.

From this viewpoint it is apparent that dealing with problems of violence involves a basically cyclical process. Initial assessment of the problem gives rise to a preliminary formulation according to which the behaviour "makes sense". On the basis of such a formulation an intervention procedure may be developed together with a strategy for its assessment. According to this assessment the intervention will be seen as either successful or a failure. If the former, the problem is solved and no further action need to be taken. If the latter, more information is available on which to develop further or change a formulation and try again. The various steps may therefore be summarised as follows:

1. Gather all possible potentially useful information regarding the problem.

2. On the basis of the information available devise a formulation which accounts for all the available information.

3. On the basis of this formulation devise an intervention programme and associated assessment procedures.

4. On the basis of the assessment decide (a) whether the intervention actually took place and (b) whether or not it was successful.

5. If not successful and the intervention did take place, revise the formulation in the light of this new information and return to stage 3 above.

The cycle of stages 3, 4 and 5 can therefore be continued until the problem is solved, each cycle providing more and more information about the problem and hence increasing the knowledge on which the formulation is based. The more information there exists regarding a formulation the more likely it is to be correct. Using such a strategy, attempts need only be discontinued when either the formulation appears to be correct but nothing can be done to alter the relevant processes, or when all conceivable formulations have proved inadequate. Such circumstances will occur only rarely, and more commonly persistence will result in success.

PRACTICAL IMPLICATIONS

It is important that procedures used for dealing with violence are, as far as possible, carefully evaluated. Such evaluation can however be more difficult than might be imagined, and a systematic approach to evaluation may involve the following:

1. Wherever possible in dealing with individuals information should be gathered regarding the baseline level of aggression. Such a measure may not always be possible however since violence may be an infrequent or in some cases a "once only" behaviour. Additionally the need to take urgent action may preclude the gathering of baseline data.

2. The use of reversal procedures (e.g. ABAB designs) will similarly be inappropriate in many cases, a return to baseline levels of aggression being undesirable or even dangerous. Some of the problems may be avoided by the use of multiple baseline designs, in particular when the multiple baseline is across the subjects rather than the behaviours.

3. Evaluation may also be done at the level of the group rather than the level of the individual. Typically this will involve dividing potential groups of subjects into comparable subgroups and treating them in an identical manner except with respect to the treatment to be evaluated. Should the outcome be different over the various groups this supports the notion that the treatment does indeed have an effect.

4. Often the aim of an intervention will not be to reduce the violence shown by an individual but rather to reduce the amount of violence encountered in particular settings. Here identifying characteristics of the setting which might account for its high level of aggression can lead to attempts to change these characteristics and resolve the problem. As with dealing with individuals, it is necessary to obtain wherever possible sound baseline data against which to compare the subsequent results.

5. Often in practice evaluation will involve indirect measures such as diaries, self reports etc. with a consequent need for caution in interpretations. The use of groups results may

involve difficulties in generalising from the average effect on a group to the specific effect on an individual. Interpretation of such data as follow-up results needs to be in the context of what changes would actually be expected in the light of the intervention. Such problems mean that evaluation needs to be with careful consideration of the strengths and weaknesses of the data involved.

6. When done carefully an evaluation provides further valuable information permitting refinement of the formulation. Intervention therefore passes through a cycle of stages of evaluation, formulation, intervention and back to evaluation until a satisfactory result is obtained.

Chapter Eleven

EVALUATING RESEARCH INTO VIOLENCE

One of the few definite statements whch can be made
about violence is that it is   still   not completely
understood. As a result workers concerned with
aggression and violence still have much research to
conduct.   Unfortunately research,   however   well
conducted, is never without its problems, and it is
necessary for those who wish to keep up to date   to
be aware of the pitfalls apparent in various   areas
of research. Some of problems recur throughout
different styles of research: other problems may be
associated particularly with one or two   styles.
Whilst it would not be possible to list all   the
possible pitfalls, it is worth noting a few of   the
more commonly encountered problems.

Subject Problems
All approaches suffer to some extent from   the
difficulty of subject characteristics. Most of   the
experimental and ethological work, for   example, is
conducted with non-human subjects.   Evolutionary
theory suggests of course a degree of   continuity
between humans and other species: on the other hand
humans have a number of unique characteristics which
may necessitate caution in extending the results of
animal studies to human violence. Wherever possible
work on other species should be repeated with   human
subjects. However the nature of the subject   matter
makes it ethically impossible to directly   replicate
some of the animal work on human subjects, and often
experiments can only be replicated on humans if they
are considerably toned down: the electric shock   of
an animal experiment may be replaced by a   harsh
criticism from an   experimenter,   for   example.
Similarly the aggression itself may be exhibited   in
only a mild form compared to the animal experiments,

for example telling stories with a higher violence content on a projective test, or hitting a life-size rubber doll. All of these raise the problem of the extent to which the stimuli or responses in question adequately represent those in normal aggressive episodes. The problem of extending animal work is of course particularly acute when dealing with such effects as hormonal variation: as described in Chapter Three, for example, there is not even consistency across non-human species in their response to physiological change. The effect of castration on the aggression of rodents is not the same as its effect on the aggression of dogs. In such circumstances it becomes particularly problematic to extend the results of such work to humans.

Even when dealing with human subjects there are problems. The stimuli and responses which can ethically be used with normal subjects run the risk of being unrealistic. If we choose to study those individuals who are, in reality, violent, we often run the risk of having to deal with a highly selected group who may not give results comparable to a wider population. Studying violent individuals in prisons, for example, restricts us to studying only those whose violence has resulted in imprisonment: it will be hard to know the extent to which the results will also apply to those whose violence does not result in imprisonment (e.g. the perpetrators of much domestic violence). When looking at the effect of neurological disturbance on violence in humans it is inevitable that the damage will have involved a number of complicating factors not apparent in the animal laboratory. Thus the individual whose violence is associated with temporal lobe damage following a road traffic accident might also, in the same accident, have lost friends or family members. It will be difficult under such circumstances to know to what extent the violence is a result of the brain damage rather than resentment or self-recrimination regarding the accident, or even such results as the loss of a driving licence.

Little if any research is conducted on samples which truly represent the aggressive members of the human race. In interpreting such research we are forced to choose one of two options: either to assume that the results will apply generally despite the biased nature of the sample, or to limit generalisations to that subset of the population which the sample can without doubt be claimed to

161

represent. In practice the usual course of action falls somewhere between these extremes, and the individual scientist will judge to what extent the limitations of the sample restrict the generality of the results. Such a judgement will be based on such issues as the current state of knowledge regarding the importance of the selection factors, the compatibility or otherwise of the results obtained with the existing body of knowledge and so on. In the final analysis however any such judgement will be a matter of opinion, and it is important that opinion not be confused with fact.

Problems with Causality

Much research encounters difficulties in identifying with confidence what are the important causal factors in a phenomenon. Thus an undercontrolled individual may become frequently involved in fights: over a period of time such fighting may result in brain damage. Subsequent study of such individuals would find an association between brain damage and frequent fighting but would be unable to say whether the brain damage caused the aggression or vice versa: without being able to follow the process through from the beginning the direction of causality woould be impossible to determine. By the same logic it may be difficult to determine whether an undercontrolled personality caused the frequent fighting or whether repeated experience of possibly successful fighting caused the individual to become undercontrolled.

To some extent these problems are overcome by experimental methods where manipulation of some relevant variable can allow subsequent fluctuations in another to be monitored. Thus removing a reinforcer successively from different types of aggressive behaviour shown by an individual implies a definite direction of causation if successful: since the therapist or experimenter controls the reinforcers it follows that it can only be the variations in reinforcement which produce the variations in aggression rather than vice versa. It is important however, even in experimental work, that such issues be considered carefully and that directions of causality be explicitly checked rather than merely assumed.

A related problem concerns what may be called the "grass is green" argument. The difficulty is of the following form: if I assert that every blade of grass I've found is green, this does not prove that

all green things are therefore grass - they may be
paints, motor cars, fabrics etc. Similarly if I
discover that most extremely aggressive people are
overcontrolled this does not mean that most
overcontrolled people may become extremely
aggressive. This problem is of course common in
dealing with specific groups of violent individuals:
were I to discover that most murderers are
husbands, it would not follow that most husbands are
murderers. To know this it would be necessary to
look at husbands and see how many were murderers,
not to look at murderers and see how many are
husbands.

This problem is only partly solved by the use of
control groups. If, for example, I were to find
that overcontrolled individuals occurred twice as
often in groups of violent offenders than in the
general population this may still mean nothing more
than that, say, 60% of violent individuals are
overcontrolled by comparison with 30% of non-violent
individuals. If we assume that there are, say, a
hundred times as many non-violent individuals in
society as there are violent, this means that there
are still fifty times as many non-violent
overcontrolled individuals as violent overcontrolled
individuals.

Finally, a general problem should be noted which
comes under the broad heading of "expectancy
effects". Basically this refers to the observation
that individual perceptions may be affected quite
substantially by what the person expects to
perceive: the problem is particularly acute when
the observations are vague. Thus if asked to assess
the degree of violence apparent in children's
stories, a person will be likely to see as more
violent those said to come from aggressive children
than those said to come from non-aggressive
children. Thus, particularly when the judgements to
be made are highly subjective, it is important to
guard against biasing these judgements by providing
clues about what to expect. It should be noted that
an aspect of this can also affect the subjects
themselves. This "placebo effect" has been of
particular importance in drug studies, since it was
found that subjects would report a number of
apparently physiological changes even when given
preparations which were pharmacologically inert. As
a result it is common for drug research to be
conducted according to a "double-blind" procedure,
where neither the subject nor the person assessing
the effects knows whther the drug was real or an

inert placebo. Even in animal research a "single blind" procedure is considered preferable, experimenters who evaluate the effects of drugs remaining, until after the assessment, ignorant about which animals received which preparation. Analogous procedures have been adopted in other fields (e.g. in the evaluation of psychological treatments) but are not usually practical in such areas as ethology and anthropology. In consequence the evaluation of research in such areas must take into account the possibility that the results are influenced by expectancy effects.

In addition to these general problems, each of the areas conributing to violence research has its own characteristic problems. Included amongst these might be the following:

Problems of Biological Research
In addition to the general problems mentioned above, biological research presents a number of particular problems. Physical biology has a number of specific difficulties. ESB studies, (see Chapter Three) for example, present a number of technological difficulties. These include accuracy of placement of electrodes, which may in fact not reach the area of the brain for which they are destined, a fact which may only be established at post-mortem. Even when electrodes are precisely located, the effects obtained may be sensitive to various parameters of the stimulation such as the intensity and frequency of the current. Often this renders difficult the interpretation of the results, since there is a risk that the more intense the stimulation, the more likely it is that surrounding brain tissues will also be stimulated, confusing the results. At the very least such difficulties render problematic the possibility of applying the results in clinical practice.

In a similar vein, drug research raises a number of problems since, like ESB, drug effects are often sensitive to a number of parameters. Thus drugs may, by varying the dose, come to have quite different effects on behaviour: a drug which stimulates behaviour at one dose may suppress it at another. Since the body adapts to most drugs, and does so at a varying rate, this makes reliance on drugs to produce anything but the most crude of effects somewhat hazardous. In evaluating research on drugs it is important to ensure that such factors as dose-response curves, duration of action, long term follow-up and possible side effects are reported. Similarly although the need for double-blind studies is now generally accepted in the evaluation of drugs, claims are sometimes made for drug effectiveness on the basis of studies which do not meet such a definition.

It is also important to remember that the body will often react to a drug in such a way as to counteract its effects. It is necessary therefore to monitor the effects of the drug over a continued period. Where it is not intended that a drug be used continuously, assessment should be made of the chances of a "rebound" effect when the drug is discontinued, the subject's condition on withdrawal possibly being worse than when originally prescribed.

With respect to genetic factors it is important to note that association in the clinic between some inherited problem and violence does not necessarily establish a causal link. The XYY individuals in Special Hospitals, for example, are probably quite unrepresentative of XYY individuals as a whole. To establish that the XYY pattern leads to violence the appropriate question is not "how many violent people are XYY" but rather "how many XYY people are violent".

A number of other problems also occur in biological research, such as the difficulties of obtaining reliable assays of certain hormones, the problems of unwanted side-effects of drugs (which may only appear after some considerable time). At the very least, assessment of any biological research should consider the following basic questions:

(1) Has the study been well conducted, e.g. meeting double-blind or single-blind criteria as appropriate?

(2) Is consideration given to such issues as the technological problems, e.g. electrode placement, stimulation parameters?

(3) Where a link has been drawn between a clinical condition (e.g. Temporal lobe epilepsy) and violence, had consideration been given to the (usually large) numbers of people with the condition who are not violent?

(4) If the study involves treatment, has consideration been given to the effects of prolonged treatment, both in terms of the continued usefulness of the treatment and the risk of possible side-effects?

(5) In ethological studies, in particular, do

the subjects and settings studied adequately represent those of practical interest? An ethological study of aggression in the limpet is unlikely to have much relevance to everyday human aggression.

Obviously not all of these questions will apply to any given study. Moreover particular studies may give rise to their own specific problem areas, and increasing expertise in such areas will require greater sophistication of questioning.

Problems of Sociological and Anthropological Research

By and large, sociological and anthropological research is conducted with human subjects and involves little if any biological manipulation. Some subject problems remain, however. In many anthropological studies the typicality of the subjects may be open to question, especially where these subjects form a subsection of a larger culture (e.g. street gangs) since it is then necessary to determine what caused those individuals to join the subculture. It could be argued, for example, that some other factor caused the individuals to become aggressive, whereupon such individuals sought out other like-minded people, thereby forming a gang. Under such circumstances the aggression would perhaps be better described as the cause of the gang subculture than its consequence. More commonly the two will interact and questions of cause and effect will appear too simplistic.

In the study of simple cultures the anthropologist must guard against concluding that violence is not apparent in a society simply on the basis that it was not observed. It may be, for example, that violence has become ritualised and occurs only at rare, special festivals. Or the violence may be present, but considered somewhat shameful and concealed from the anthropologist. The skilled worker will consider these possibilities and investigate them, but the careless or unskilled researcher may not.

In general, however, most anthropologists are well aware of these danger areas and make every effort to avoid them. Rather less easy to avoid in such work are the difficulties in identifying the relevant causal factors influencing the amount of violence. It is one thing to note that the Hopi culture discourages violence, but quite another to identify which aspects of the culture are responsible. Often the best that can be done here is to exclude certain factors from consideration. Sipes (1973), for example, provided a telling argument against the notion that non-violence was associated with "alternative outlets" by showing that the incidence of competitive sports ran parallel to the incidence of violence. Under the supposition that such sports provide an "outlet" for aggression the opposite would have been expected. Such studies allow possible factors to be more or less convincingly eliminated, but do not necessarily allow others to be implicated.

More sociologically oriented studies also have their problems. The increased numerical emphasis common in sociology permits a much greater degree of precision than the non-numerical approaches typical of anthropology, but the numbers need to be treated with caution. Changes over time or across cultures may make dramatic differences to the apparent incidence of violence and related factors. If for example it was intended to look at relationships between suicide and homicide in different societies it would make little sense to compare the United Kingdom and Japan: in the former, suicide is still stigmatised, and for a suicide verdict to be given the evidence needs to be particularly strong, whereas in the latter suicide is part of a tradition of honour and a much more likely verdict. Differences in reported suicides may not therefore reflect true differences in the rate of suicide.

Related to this is the problem of adequate operationalisation of variables. As mentioned in Chapter One such categories as "offences against the person" may contain a number of offences which were arguably non-violent. In considering studies which use such figures it is important to consider exactly how well the measures used correspond to the problem of interest.

In considering sociological and anthropological work therefore the following questions should be considered:

(1) To what extent do the people studied have relevance to the wider population? In considering subcultures, do the members of this subculture have any common characteristic which might explain their violence?

(2) Is the researcher's degree of acceptance sufficient to permit observation of any violence, or is there a risk that violence was kept hidden?

(3) Is due consideration given to establishing causality? Since most such studies are

correlational, cause and effect can often be hard to distinguish.

(4) Is it clear exactly what the variables mean, and is their meaning exactly what is required? Reported crimes of violence, for example, will not necessarily correspond to the actual amount of violence in society.

Problems of Psychological Research

The experimental emphasis in psychology has done much to avoid the causality problems of other approaches. By directly manipulating variables and observing the effects of such manipulations, the direction of causality can often be clearly demonstrated. Psychological work is not, however, without its problems. The range of approaches used within psychology implies the possibility of a number of problems but also of the problems of one approach being avoided by the strengths of another.

Thus studies of personality types and aggression suffer in much the same way as anthropological and biological studies. Being correlational they leave open the question of causation, and dealing with a particular (violent) subgroup they often fail to consider the large number of people with the same personality characteristics who are not aggressive. In principle however it is possible to conceive of a treatment which had direct influence on the personality, e.g. the modification of undercontrol by assertion training. Changes in violence resulting from change in personality do much to clarify the question of causal direction.

Experimental approaches are not without their problems however. Psychology in particular has been dominated by the use of statistical procedures in assessing the results of experiments. In a typical experiment subjects will be randomly assigned to two groups, an "experimental" group who may for example receive some treatment and a "control" group who may receive no treatment (or a treatment with what is felt to be the vital ingredient missing). Since both groups will be affected similarly by external factors (e.g. a TV campaign against violence) the only difference will be that one has had the treatment. Any differences between the two groups in the end, therefore, may only be due to the treatment ingredient. (The logic is of course flawed in that the treatment may interact into extraneous factors, e.g. a treatment which consists of being told to watch TV will only result in a difference if there are relevant TV programmes. If such programmes are being shown the "treatment" will appear to be effective: if not it will appear ineffective. In general however the likelihood of such fortuitous interactions is felt to be low.)

In such studies the criterion for deciding on effectiveness is the extent to which the difference between the average of the two groups is greater than would be expected by chance: such results are said to be "statistically significant". (Similar procedures are used in much biological research, where similar problems apply.) It is important to note that statistical significance implies only that a treatment is not totally ineffective, not that its effects are substantial. A distinction has therefore to be drawn between results which are statistically and clinically significant, since the two are not synomynous. A treatment which reduced aggressive outbursts to 95% of the original frequency may have little clinical significance: yet it is not totally ineffective, and research on the treatment may consistently give results which are statistically significant. To add to the confusion, it is also possible to obtain results which are clinically significant but not statistically significant (Owens 1979). Results moreover may show that a given treatment is useful on average whilst still being ineffective as far as some of the group members are concerned. That is to say, results which apply to the group cannot necessarily be generalised to the individual.

In response to these problems a number of studies have concentrated on demonstrating treatment effectiveness directly without the use of complex statistics, and reporting the results of individual subjects rather than groups. Whilst such studies are easy to interpret in themselves, extension of the results to other individuals and settings depends on a good understanding of the processes involved in order that the effect of a change of subject or situation can be predicted. Establishment of such generalisability usually depends upon the results being successfully repeated with a range of individuals and settings, a process known as replication. Without adequate replication, studies of small numbers of individuals need to be interpreted with caution.

Obviously, since much psychological research is conducted with non-human species, there arises a question of the extent to which such studies provide an adequate analogue of human violence. In general psychologists have tended to replicate their animal results, where possible, with comparable human experiments: where this is not (e.g. for ethical reasons) practical, the results are replicated over a wide range of other species. Whilst obviously less satisfactory, such a procedure does provide some basis for increased confidence in the applicability of the results to humans

Much psychological research is of course non-experimental, as, for example, when groups of subjects are surveyed in order to detect differences in such things as personality characteristics. The identification of personality characteristics however carries its own problems. It is, of course, as with biological work, necessary also to consider the large number of individuals who share the characteristic but who are not actually violent. From a technological viewpoint, also, such studies have problems: a personality test which is of high effectiveness in distinguishing a group of known violent individuals from non-violent ones, may actually be counter-productive when applied to a wider population where the overall proportion of violent individuals is much less than in the validation sample. This problem, known as the "base rate" problem, is too complex for consideration in detail. It can be shown that a test which, when used, permits more accurate classification of individuals roughly equally distributed in a population, can actually increase the number of errors made when later applied to a population where the individuals in question are either relatively rare or extremely common (for a fuller discussion see Owens 1984). That is to say, a test may be useful in detecting violent individuals in one population and, without any change to the test, result in greater numbers of errors when applied to a different population. In practice this means at the very least that newly published tests claiming to distinguish violent from non-violent individuals should be carefully checked. The proportions of violent and non-violent individuals in the original sample on which the test was validated should as closely as possible approximate those in the population to which the test is to be applied.

The non-technological aspects of personality research, too, have their problems. Much research, for example, has gone into investigating the extent to which personality characteristics associated with aggression are inherited and the extent to which they are learned. The question cannot simply be answered by looking at how similar parents are to their children, since the likelihood exists that, to some extent at least, parents will bring up their children to conform to the standards they themselves hold. Nor can it be solved by simply comparing the similarity between adopted and natural children with their parents, since adopted children, even when young, have already had a number of experiences different to their new siblings. Moreover the fact that the parents, and often the children themselves, know them to be adopted may itself produce substantial effects.

It has been argued that the study of identical twins raised apart may provide a solution, using the following logic. Personality, it is said, is a result of the combination of heredity and environment. If one of these can be held constant without affecting the other, their relative contributions can be assessed. Identical twins have the same genes and any differences between them must therefore be caused by the environment. As mentioned above, this observation is unhelpful in most cases since the twins, besides having identical genes, will also have similar environments; an estimate of the contribution made by heredity in general will be an underestimate, since the similarity of their environment reduces this effect. If, however, the twins are raised apart, the argument goes, their environments will vary as much as any other two unrelated children; reduction in the differences between them must therefore be due to the similarity of their genetic make-up, providing a way of assessing the relative contributions of genetics and environment. If identical twins raised apart are more similar than other unrelated children, this implies that the genetic similarity must be responsible.

Unfortunately the practice is rather more complex; identical twins raised apart are relatively uncommon so that only small samples can be obtained; statistically this implies increased scope for error. The scarcity of such individuals means that it is rare for studies to be replicated; since the exposure of Cyril Burt as having falsified early data of this nature, people have become naturally suspicious of unreplicated reports in this field.

There is an additional problem in the consideration of the environments of the raised-apart twins, in that the similarity of such environments for the twins is still likely to be

171

greater than the similarity of environments for
children in the population at large; the homes of
fostered identical twins are unlikely to encompass
the range of environments found in the world at
large, from a Glasgow tenement to a royal palace.
Since the environments to which the children go are
likely to be similar, one would expect the twins to
show similarity even if the contribution of genetic
factors were negligible. Estimates of heritability
based on such studies are likely to be
correspondingly inflated. Without some objective
measure of "similarity of environment" it is
impossible to allow for this, hence rendering
meaningless precise estimates of heritability.

A number of other problems widespread throughout
research on violence occur frequently within
psychological work. In particular psychological
research may often involve measures of aggression
which are open to suspicion: amongst the measures
which psychologists have used are stories told in
response to Thematic Apperception Test pictures,
ratings of one's own feelings of hostility and even
the sounding of motor car horns. Obviously some
caution must be exercised in assuming equivalence in
the sounding of a car horn and the wielding of a
meat cleaver by an angry spouse.

In considering psychological research, then, the
following questions might usefully be involved in
evaluation:-

(1) Do results which are reported as being of
statistical significance also represent results of
clinical significance?

(2) Are results obtained for the group in
general capable of being extended to particular
individuals?

(3) In non-statistical designs, are the
subjects and problems sufficiently similar to others
to permit generalisation? To what extent have the
results actually been replicated with other subjects
and settings?

(4) Where studies purport to present tests
distinguishing aggressive from non-aggressive
individuals, do the base rates in the samples on
which the test was established match those in the
population on which it is to be used?

(5) In studies of heritability, is excessive
faith placed on the estimates of environmental
determination on which the heritability estimates
are based?

(6) Do the measures of aggression adequately
represent the aggressive behaviour in which we are

actually interested?

Obviously the differences between different approaches are not so clear-cut that the questions suggested for evaluation of one approach will never be applicable to another. Equally obviously a number of other questions will often be relevant, depending upon the specific interests of the questioner and the details of the study.

Few research studies will pass all of the above questions without difficulty. This is not to say, of course, that studies which are found to have problems should be rejected: to do so would be to reject almost the whole of systematic research into violence. Rather it is necessary to consider such issues in order tht the information provided by research be placed in its proper perspective. To reject research is no answer, since non-systematic approaches fare much worse than systematic research when faced with the above questions.

By placing research into its proper perspective it is possible to treat results with a degree of circumspection. Few if any studies will provide conclusive evidence regarding some questions. Rather it is necessary to take the results of various studies, to evaluate each individually, and to attempt to integrate those into a total picture. Sometimes the conclusions of a study will fit neatly into the total picture, but this is not to say that they are necessarily correct or that the overall theory is true: conversely, evidence which seems not to fit need not imply that the theory is wrong. In each case a decision has to be made as to whether a study is basically sound, with whatever that implies for a theory, or whether the study is faulty. Few theories are so well supported that they cannot be open to doubt: the stronger the evidence in favour of a theory, the stronger will a study have to be to cast doubt upon it. Conversely the better-designed a study, the more appropriate it will be to modify the theory.

Of course it makes sense to consider studies not individually but with respect to each other. Thus two studies may each have faults, but the faults of each may be remedied by the other. Or a possible failing of one study may be clarified by a subsequent study. Thus an initial study may demonstrate reactive aggression in rats. Such a study may be considered of little significance by a reader who fels that the results would have been different with human subjects. When a subsequent study replicates the work (or part of it) with humans, the same reader may than be more inclined to go back to the original study and reconsider its results.

What is required then is a skilled and reasoned evaluation of research evidence. The fact that no study is perfect should not blind the reader to the fact that some are better than others. To know not only which studies are better than others, but also to be able to assess the strengths and weaknesses of each, is a necessary skill in keeping up to date with research. With such skills it is possible not only to compare alternative theories, by comparing the quality of the evidence in support of them, but also to modify such comparisons as further evidence becomes available.

PRACTICAL IMPLICATIONS

In our present state of knowledge it is essential that those working in potentially violent settings be able to keep up to date with findings in the research literature. Whilst such literature commonly constitutes the best available information on violence, it is by no means without its problems. The individual reading research material should ask a number of questions including;

1. Does the specific choice of subject affect the validity of the results? Put another way, the question involves deciding whether or not the subjects in the study adequately represent the individuals to whom the results are to be extended. Note that to decide this already presupposes some knowledge of what is important in aggression. In some respects a rat may provide a useful representation of human aggression (e.g. in its behaviour during extinction). In other respects it may be quite unrepresentative (e.g. in the effects of certain hormones). It is important also, when subjects in a study are aggressive individuals, to ask what is known of similar non-aggressive individuals.

2. Is it clear what is cause and what is effect? Often certain characteristics will coincide without one actually being the cause of the other: for example a hormone level may change at the same time as behaviour changes, but both be independent consequences of some external event. Often causality is assumed on intuitive grounds, a particularly hazardous procedure. Whilst it may, for example, seem obvious that hormonal change causes behavioural change, rather than vice versa, evidence suggests that the converse is equally likely.

3. Has the study adequately controlled for extraneous factors? Important here are such effects as placebo effects, expectancy effects and so on: often studies will need to fulfil "double-blind" criteria in order to do so. Similarly it may be necessary to check for technological problems e.g. changes in drug effects with changes of dose. Each particular area of research may appropriately be considered in the light of the specific questions asked in the body of Chapter Eleven.

Inevitably few research studies will be found to be flawless if subjected to this level of questioning. Such studies should not be completely rejected because of the flaws revealed. Rather they should be considered in the light of their limitations, care being taken not to rely excessively on any single piece of research. Often the flaws of one study will be compensated for by the strengths of another. Under such circumstances it is possible to develop an increased confidence in particular conclusions.

Chapter Twelve

TOWARDS A LESS VIOLENT FUTURE

Whilst the development of procedures for dealing
with violence is obviously of value, it would
clearly be preferable if such procedures were
unnecessary, that is, if violence were prevented in
the first place. The possibility of non-violence
certainly exists, as seen in anthropological
studies: human beings are capable of co-existing
peacefully. Exactly how to achieve such
non-violence is however far from clear. Moreover it
is difficult to determine an appropriate balance
between taking action which is urgently needed and
awaiting the clearer understanding which further
research may bring.

There seems little doubt that in the past
attempts at reducing societal violence have been
proposed in advance of the requisite empirical
information. Much opinion for example has suggested
procedures of either catharsis or displacement for
the reduction of violence. Such function, it has
been suggested, may be served by the space race, the
Olympic Games and so forth. In a therapeutic
setting procedures aimed at "discharging aggressive
energy" may have the effect of making the individual
feel better, but the major effect of this seems to
be the reinforcement of such behaviour making it
more likely in the future. Similarly, empirical
test of the effects of competitive sport suggest
that such activities are likely to foster, rather
than reduce, aggression (Zillman et al., 1978). In
a critical review of the catharsis/displacement
literature Zillman (1979) concluded that such an
approach to the reduction of aggression was futile
and that other approaches were necessary.

THE PREVENTION OF VIOLENCE

On a moment's reflection it is perhaps obvious that a complex problem like violence could not be prevented in any simple way. Indeed there is the risk that attempts at simple solutions may, even if successful at reducing one form of violence, be counter-productive in dealing with another. In considering the reduction of violence, therefore, it is perhaps helpful to look separately at the different processes and factors involved.

Reactive Aggression

It is perhaps ironic that whilst the socialisation and education of people in Western society involves the acquisition of much knowledge regarding the occurence of violence, little if any systematic effort is made to teach them to handle potentially violent situations in which they find themselves. Lessons in history recount the details of hundreds of years of warfare: television, films and the like present models for dealing with problems by recourse to violence. Yet when confronted with the kinds of aversive events which elicit reactive aggression, self-control on the part of the individual becomes essential if violence is to be avoided. Since it seems unlikely that aversive events can be completely eliminated from an individual's life, some skill in handling such events in a non-violent way is likely to be beneficial. The kinds of procedure used in dealing with reactive aggression in therapy could, to a large extent, be taught to the wider population, as an "educational" rather than a "therapeutic" exercise (the parallels between learning and therapy have of course been made before e.g. Skinner 1953, Rogers 1960, Kelly 1955). In this way the individual may be taught both to prepare for aversive situations, to rehearse positive solutions and to exert self-control when in such situations. Since the individual is often insensitive to external factors when in such situations, it follows that an approach based on self-control skills is more likely to succeed than ones based on such factors as the threat of punishment.

Of course, to say that aversive events cannot be completely eliminated is not to say that they cannot be reduced. Indeed since the kinds of events with which reactive aggression is associated tend to be interpersonal, it follows that a change in the way people interact may produce a corresponding change in the extent to which they elicit aggression from each other. In particular it appears that much of society's violence, that which occurs within families or between individuals known to each other, may be avoided if the people concerned become more sensitive to the reactions of others. Where a violent reaction occurs in response to prolonged irritation, it seems likely that taking action to stop such irritation before it produces uncontrollable reactions may alleviate interpersonal violence. This is of course the strategy implicit in such procedures as assertion training. It should be noted however that such skills rely for their continued use on a sucessful outcome. Even the most highly skilled assertion will be valueless in the face of a marriage partner who refuses to concede in any way. For such procedures as assertion training to reach their full potential, therefore, it may well be necessary to avoid the gross power imbalances which occur in many relationships. At present such relationships as marriage often leave one partner in a much more powerful position vis-a-vis the other. A husband may be physically stronger, may have access to finance etc. Where such imbalances can be avoided, steps should be taken to do so: where not, other action should be taken to compensate. For the foreseeable future men are likely, in general, to be physically stronger than women: since women are unlikely to be able to compete physically, the need for a place of escape (e.g. the Battered Wive's Refuge) may be crucial. Legal support too may be needed: only recently has the possibility that a man could be convicted of raping his wife begun to be taken seriously.

In dealing with reactive aggression, then, action on two distinct fronts may be necessary. In the first place conditions must be as favourable as possible for the prevention of eliciting situations: where power relationships are equal and one partner is unable to succeed in a struggle for dominance, then the alternative strategy of cooperation becomes more likely. Where aversive situations are unavoidable, increased skill in preparing for, and dealing with, them reduces the possibility of a violent outcome.

Operant Aggression
In dealing with operant aggression, the picture is somewhat different. Violence in society has a

number of reinforcers and it seems likely that as long as violence provides an efficient access to such reinforcers it will continue to occur. Certainly with respect to some of the most obvious reinforcers violence continues for many to be the only practical route to their acquisition. The notion of equality of opportunity is in many Western societies nothing more than a myth. The working class child from the slums, who spends over twenty years in education and becomes, say, a successful physician or a professor, is still likely to earn a yearly salary which amounts to less than an aristocrat, born into wealth, spends on a new car or a coming-out party. Since most people fail to reach even the financial position of the physician or professor but will be faced with the prospect of spending their lives in much more difficult settings, it is hard to be surprised when violence is chosen as the only practical means of access to wealth. Indeed such an approach may be seen by the individual as morally, as well as practically, defensible: no other way of obtaining an equitable share of society's wealth may be apparent. Whether a completely equitable distribution of wealth is practical or essential, some steps towards equality may be appropriate. In the United Kingdom, for example, the Inland Revnue estimates that over half the nation's wealth is owned by only 5% of the population. Since most of this wealth is unearned, being inherited or interest on capital, it is hard not to sympathise with those who claim it to be unjust. When one person can spend twice as much on a fur coat as the average annual income, inequality may be said to be extreme.

The avoidance of operant aggression involves a society in which access to reinforcers is easier through non-violent means than through violent ones. In many societies the chances of success using non-violent methods (gambling, becoming a pop star etc.) are so remote as to be negligible: for every one who suceeds hundreds fall by the wayside. If operant violence is to be eliminated, much greater access to reinforcers like money must be available through productive socially useful activities rather than through violence.

This is not to say, of course, that to produce a society in which all had equal wealth would be to produce a non-violent society (though it is likely to be a necessary precondition for such a society). Many other reinforcers serve to maintain operant aggression: the prestige of the war hero, the

masculinity of the fighter. A radical rethink of
the value society attaches to such behaviour may be
necessary, such that status and prestige are
accorded on the basis of more constructive and
socially useful behaviour than assaulting another
person or shooting a teenage boy who happens to be
in an opposing army. Unless a higher value is set
on compassionate, kindly and cooperative behaviour a
reduction in the cruel and competitive cannot be
expected.

Of course, as with reactive aggression, it seems
unlikely that society could be so constructed that
positive behaviour was always, for all individuals,
more likely to lead to reinforcement than violent
behaviour. One possible solution to this has been
considered by Zillman (1979) who advocates the use
of punishment as a means of controlling operant
aggression. Certainly for the violence which
remains when all other preventative measures have
been taken the use of punishment may have a valuable
role. Currently punishment seems to be largely
ineffective as a controller of violent behaviour
despite the calls for longer and more severe prison
sentences. Possibly this is due in part to the fact
that a violent offence, at the moment, has a
reasonable change of going unpunished. Even of
violent crimes reported to the police a sizeable
number (some 20% in the United Kingdom) do not
result in a prosecution. Many more violent
offences, it appears, may go unreported (e.g. much
family violence). At present, then, punishment may
be relatively ineffective, in part because people
see a realistic chance of "getting away with it".

It is possible however that if those charged
with dealing with violent crime (typically the
police) had less to deal with, then their success
rate with the violence remaining would increase.
That is to say if most violence were eliminated by
means of the kinds of social and political change
outlined earlier, that which remained might be
within the power of the authorities to control.

Reducing the level of violent crime to a low
level would also make it possible to provide
realistic rehabilitative measures. If reinforcement
could be obtained through positive behaviour in a
more equitable society, those imprisoned would have
good cause to learn such positive behaviours. Under
such conditions motivation to participate in
rehabilitative schemes would be higher since they
would offer a chance for the offender to return to
society and to share equally in society's wealth.

Such access to a fair share of the society's wealth is unlikely under the present system of teaching prisoners such skills as the use of a sewing machine.

Under the right conditions of social and political change, then, it is possible that most violence could be prevented, with that remaining being susceptible to control by punishment. As regards the latter, such control, once established, would be likely to have its effects amplified by positive feedback. Thus reducing the level of violence would increase the chance that violent acts which did occur would be punished. Such an increased risk of punishment would result in a further decrease in the rate of violence, resulting in even higher risk of punishment and so forth. In a similar way the increased resources for rehabilitation would make such procedures more likely to be successful, which would free further resources, making future programmes even better, and so on. Thus once violence had been brought to a manageable level by societal change, the remaining violence could be susceptible to "mopping up" by punishment and constructive rehabilitation measures.

Problems of Controlling Violence

As a final note it is worth remembering that the control of violence is not always a desirable aim. One of the reasons for suspicion regarding surgical, chemical and electrical approaches to the control of violence is the risk such procedures present of subsequent exploitation. Skinner (1971) has discussed at length the notion of "countercontrol". Lack of exploitation of one group by another is most common when each group is capable of exerting control over the other. Where countercontrol is absent, Skinner points out, is where abuse and exploitation are most commonly found. Thus children, the mentally handicapped, the psychotic, the elderly and other powerless groups are often found to be the victims of one form or another of social cruelty. In producing a peaceful society, it is not necessarily desirable to produce a placid one, incapable of revolt against exploitation.

A number of writers (e.g. Vadya 1961, Coser 1967) have pointed to the functional value of aggressive conflict in various societies. The evidence of history seems to suggest that those in power will rarely sacrifice such power willingly, and that violence is often the only way in which freedom has been obtained. Even where such freedom seems to have been obtained through non-violence the threat of violence may be involved. The liberation of India by Ghandi is often cited as an example of the success of non-violence, yet it is far from clear that his efforts would have succeeded had there not at the same time been a threat of a communist takeover, an outcome which would have been even less desirable from the point of view of the British rulers. Only under such circumstances did those in power relent, regarding Ghandi as the lesser of two evils.

The control of violence, then, ideally requires the elimination of violence by the elimination of the functions that it serves. It is perhaps in this respect that the social and psychological are preferable to the medical and technological. By dealing with the reasons for violence there is the potential for a peaceful society, but one which is still capable of the use of violence in defending itself against exploitation.

PRACTICAL IMPLICATIONS

Obviously any attempt at eliminating violence from society must involve a number of measures. Some of these will be effective in dealing with operant aggression, some with reactive, and some with both. In most cases only fairly general guidelines may be offered for reducing societal violence. These include:

1. The notion that alternative outlets will provide a substitute for violence seems not to be supported by either historical, anthropological or psychological research. Indeed, if anything, the results of such studies tend to imply that activities like violent sport go hand in hand with violence in society.

2. Opportunity should be available as far as possible for people to remove sources of irritation (stimuli for reactive aggression) from their lives without recourse to violent measures. For skills such as assertion to be effective in doing so it is important to eliminate the gross power imbalances implicit in many relationships. In addition it may be important to ensure that where such stimuli cannot be eliminated (e.g. an intractable spouse) then adequate opportunity is provided for escape.

3. Reinforcement of aggression occurs at a high level in many societies. As long as such reinforcers are available for aggressive behaviour it should occasion no surprise that the behaviour continues. When the probability of reinforcement through aggression is compared with the probability of reinforcement through non-aggressive activities we see that not only does society provide reinforcement for aggression but that for many people aggression is the only practical route to reinforcement.

4. If it were possible to reduce the incidence of violence by measures such as those described above, it is possible that some measures which are largely ineffective at the present time may become of value. With less violence to deal with in society such procedures as punishment and rehabilitation might become available for all violent offenders. If successful, this would create a positive feedback with less violence and therefore even more successful rehabilitation.

184

5. It is important however that, where violence is to be eliminated, this is not done at the cost of creating a passive unresisting populace. Historically the elimination of political abuse has almost always involved violent action. It is important that elimination of such violence does not create the opportunity for political exploitation.

REFERENCES

Adams, D. B. (1971) 'Defence and territorial behaviour dissociated by hypothalamic lesions in the rat' Nature, 232, 573-574

Azrin, N. H. and Hutchinson, R. R. (1967) 'Conditioning of the aggressive behaviour of pigeons by a fixed-interval schedule of reinforcement' Journal of the Experimental Analysis of Behaviour, 10, 395-402

Bandura, A. (1973) 'Aggression: a social learning analysis' Prentice-Hall, New Jersey

Bandura, A., Ross, D. and Ross, S. A. (1961) 'Transmission of aggression through imitation of aggressive models' Journal of Abnormal and Social Psychology, 63, 575-582

Bandura, A. and Walters, R. H. (1959) 'Adolescent aggression' Ronald Press, New York

Berkowitz, L. and Le Page, A. (1967) 'Weapons as aggression-eliciting stimuli' Journal of Personality and Social Psychology, 7, 202-207

Bernard, L. L. (1961) 'The Misuse of the Concept of Instinct' in Birney-Teevan (eds.), Instinct, D. Van Nostrand Co., Princeton, London

Binney, V., Harkell, G. and Nixon, J. (1981) 'Leaving violent men' Women's Aid Federation/Department of Environment, London

Blackburn, R. (1968) 'Personality in relation to extreme aggression in psychiatric offenders' British Journal of Psychiatry, 114, 821-828

Blacking, J. (1983) 'The social construction of violence; towards an anthropology of peace' Unpublished MS, Queen's University of Belfast

Blackman, D. E. and Sanger, D. J. (1978) 'Contemporary research in behavioural pharmacology' Plenum, New York

References

Bolton, R. (1973) 'Aggression and hypoglycaemia
    among the Qolla: a study in psychobiological
    anthropology' Ethnology, 12, 227-255
Bowlby, J. (1958) 'The nature of the child's tie to
    his mother' International Journal of
    Psychoanalysis, 39, 350-373
Brandt, R. B. (1954) 'Hopi ethics; a theoretical
    analysis' University Press, Chicago
Brazier, M. A. B. (1967) Discussion of paper by
    B. Kaada in 'Aggression and defense: neural
    mechanisms and social patterns (Brain function
    Vol. 5)' by C. D. Clemente. and D. B. Lindsley
    (eds.) University of California Press,
    Los Angeles
Breggin, P. R. (1972) 'The return of lobotomy and
    psychosurgery' Entered by the Hon. Cornelius
    E. Gallagher into the Congressional Record,
    118, (26) February 24th, Washington
Bremer, J. (1959) 'Asexualization' Macmillan,
    New York
Brody, S. (1977) 'Screen violence and film
    censorship' Home Office Research Unit
    Report No. 40, H.M.S.O., London
Buss, A. H. (1971) 'Aggression pays' in J. L.
    Singer (ed) 'The control of aggression and
    violence' Academic Press, N.Y.
Buss, A. H., Booker, A. and Buss, E.(1972)'Firing
    a weapon and aggression' Journal of
    Personality and Social Psychology, 22,
    296-302
Carney, M. W. P. (1979) 'Management of the
    disturbed patient' Nursing Times, Nov.1,
    1896-1899
Carr, E. G. and Binkhoff, J. A. (1981) 'Self
    control' in A. P. Goldstein, E. G. Carr,
    W. S. Davidson II and Paul Wehr (eds.)
    'In Response to Aggression', Pergamon,
    New York
Casey, M. D., Blank, C. E., McLean, T. M.,
    Kohn, P., Street, D. R. K., McDougall, S. M.
    Gooder, J. and Platts, J. (1973) 'Male patients
    with chromosome abnormality in the state
    hospitals' Journal of Mental Deficiency
    Research 16, 215-256
Chagnon, N. A. "Yanomamo: the fierce people"
    Holt Rinehart and Winston, N.Y.
Clark, H.B., Rosbury, T., Baer, A.M. and Baer, D.M.
    (1973) 'Timeout as a punishing stimulus in
    continuous and intermittent schedules' Journal
    of Applied Behaviour Analysis, 6, 443-455
Coser, L. A. (1967) 'Continuities in the study of

social conflict' Free Press, New York

Delgado, J. M.R. (1967) 'Social rank and radio-stimulated aggression in monkeys' Journal of Nervous and Mental Disease, 144, 383-390

Delgado, J. M. R.(1969) 'Physical Control of the Mind' Harper and Row, New York

DeMause, L. (1975) 'Our forbears made childhood a nightmare' Psychology Today, 8, 85-88

DiGiuseppe, R. A. (1977)/'The use of behaviour modification to establish rational self-statements in children' Rational Living, 10, 18-20

Dingwall, R. (1984) 'Who is to blame anyway?' Nursing Times, April 11

Dobash, R. E. and Dobash, R. P. (1980) 'Violence against wives' Open Books, London

Doering, C. H., Brodie, H. K. H., Kraemer, H. C., Becker, H. B. and Hamburg, D. A. (1974) 'Plasma testosterone levels and psychologic measures in men over a 2-month period' in R. C. Friedman, R. M. Richat and R. L. Van De Wiele (eds.) Sex differences in behaviour, Wiley, New York

Doering, C. H., Brodie, H. K. H.,, Kraemer, H. C., Moos, R. W., Becker, H. B. and Hamburg, D. A. (1975) 'Negative affect and plasma testosterone a longitudinal human study' Psychosomatic Medicine 37, 484-491

Dollard, J., Doob, L., Miller, N., Mowrer, O. and Sears, R. (1939) 'Frustration and aggression' Yale University Press, New Haven, Connecticut

Drabman, R. and Spitalnick, R. (1973) 'Social isolation as a punishment procedure: a controlled study' Journal of Experimental Child Psychology, 16, 236-249

Elias, M. (1981) 'Serum cortisol, testosterone and testosterone binding globulin responses to competitive fighting in human males' Aggressive Behaviour, 7, 215-224

Ellis, A. (1962) 'Reason and emotion in psycho-therapy' Lyle Stuart, New York

Evans, D. R. (1970) 'Specific aggression, arousal and reciprocal inhibition therapy' The Western Psychologist, 1, 125-130

Eysenck, H. J. (1964) 'Crime and Personality' Routledge, London

Eysenck, H. J. (1983) 'Current theories of crime' in E. Karas (ed.) Current Issues in Clinical Psychology, Volume 1, Plenum, New York

Ferster, C. B. (1965) 'A functional analysis of

depression' American Psychologist, 28, 857-870

Foy, E. W., Eisler, R. M. and Pinkston, S. (1975) 'Modelled assertion in a case of explosive rages' Journal of Behaviour Therapy and Experimental Psychiatry, 6, 135-138

French, P. (1983) 'Social skills for nursing practice' Croom Helm Ltd., Kent

Friedman, S. B. and Morse, C. W. (1974) 'Child abuse: a five year follow-up of early case finding in the emergency department' Paediatrics, 54, 404-410

Gibbs, T. (1984) Views from America' Nursing Times, April 24

Gil, D. G. (1968) 'The California Pilot Study' in R. E. Helfer and C. H. Kempe (eds.) The Battered Child, University of Chicago Press

Goldstein, A. P. (1982) 'Problem-solving training'in A. P. Goldstein, E. G. Carr, W. S. Davidson II and P. Wehr (eds.) In Response to Aggression, Pergamon, New York

Gregg, G. S. and Elmer, E. (1969) 'Infant injuries: accidents or abuse?' Paediatrics, 44, 434-439

Gunn, J. C. and Fenton, G. (1969) 'Epilepsy in prisons: a diagnostic survey' British Medical Journal, 4, 326-329

Haney, C., Banks, C. and Zimbardo, P. (1973) 'Interpersonal dynamics in a stimulated prison' International Journal of Criminology and Penology, 1, 69-97

Harris, M. (1976) 'Cows, pigs, wars and witches' Fontana/Collins, London

Heider, K. (1970) 'The Dugum Dani', Wenner-Gren Foundation, Viking Fund Publications, No. 49

Heimburger, R. F. Whitlock, C. C., and Kalsbeck, J. E. (1966) "Stereotaxic amygdalotomy for epilepsy with aggressive behaviour" Journal of the American Medical Association 198, 165-169

Hersen, M. and Barlow, D. (1976) 'Single case experimental designs' Pergamon, New York

Hoghughi, M. S. and Forrest, A. R. (1970) 'Eysenck's theory of criminality' British Journal of Criminology, 10, 240-254

Homme, L. (1971) 'How to use contingency contracting in the classroom' Research Press, Illinois

Hovland, C. I. and Sears, R. R. (1940) 'Minor studies of aggression: correlation of lynchings with economic indices' Journal of Psychology, 9, 301-310

Hull, D. (1974) 'Clinical features of child abuse' in C. M. Lee (ed.) Child Abuse: a reader and sourcebook, Open University, Milton Keynes

Itil, T. M. (1981) 'Drug therapy in the management
    of aggression' in P. F. Brain and D. Benton
    (eds.) Multidisciplinary approaches to
    aggression research, Elsevier/North-Holland,
    Amsterdam

Jacobs, P. A., Price, W. H., Richmond, S. and
    Ratcliffe, R. A. W. (1971) 'Chromosome
    surveys in penal institutions and approved
    schools' Journal of Medical Genetics, 8, 49-58

Jacobson, E. (1938) 'Progressive relaxation'
    University of Chicago Press, Chicago

Kallman, F.J. (1938) 'The genetics of schizophrenia'
    Augustin, New York

Keegan, J. (1976) 'The face of battle' Jonathan
    Cape, London

Kelly, G. A. (1955) 'The psychology of personal
    constructs volumes I and II' Norton, New York

Kelly, J. F. and Hake, D. F. (1970) 'An extinction
    -induced increase in an aggressive response
    with humans' Journal of the Experimental
    Analysis of Behaviour, 14, 154-164

Kempe, C. H. (1969) 'The battered child and the
    hospital' Hospital Practice, 4, 44-57

Kempe, C. H. (1971) 'Paediatric implications of
    the battered baby syndrome' Archives of
    disease in childhood, 46, 28-37

Kempe, C. H. and Helfer, R. E. (1972) 'Innovative
    therapeutic approaches' in Kempe, C. H. and
    Helfer, R. E. (eds.) Helping the battered
    child and his family, Lippinott, Philadelphia

Kempe, R. S. and Kempe, C. H. (1978) 'Child Abuse'
    Fontana, London

Kerlinger, F. N. (1972) 'Foundations of Behavioural
    Research' Holt, Rinehart and Winston, New York

King, H. E. (1961) 'Psychological effects of
    excitation in the limbic system' in D. E. Sheer
    (ed.) Electrical Stimulation of the Brain,
    University of Texas Press, Austin, Texas

Kline, N. S. and Angst, J. (1975) 'Side effects of
    psychiatric drugs' Psychiatric Annales,
    5, 411-458

Knutson, J. F., Fordyce, D. J. and Anderson, D. J.
    (1980) 'Escalation of irritable aggression:
    control by consequences and antecedents'
    Aggressive Behaviour, 6, 347-359

Koolhaas, J. M. (1978) 'Hypothalamically induced
    intra-specific aggressive behaviour in the rat'
    Experimental Brain Research, 32, 365-375

Kranz, H. (1936) 'Lebensschicksale krinomineller
    Zwillinge' Springer, Berlin

Landholt, H. (1960) 'Die Temporallenepilepsie

und ihre Psychopathologie' Karger, Basel

Lange, J. (1929) 'Verbrechen als Schicksal, Studien an kriminellen Zwillinger' Thierme, Leipzig

Lee, C. M. (1978) 'Child abuse: a reader and sourcebook' Open University Press, Milton Keynes

Leiba, P. A. (1980) 'Management of violent patients' Nursing Times, October 2, 101-104

Llewellyn, T. C. (1981) 'Aggression and hypo-glycaemia in the Andes; another look at the evidence' Current Anthropology 22, 347-352

Lynch, M. and Roberts, J. (1978) 'Predisposing factors within the family' in V. Carver (ed.) Child Abuse: a study text' Open University Press, Milton Keynes

Madsen, C. H., Becker, W. C. and Thomas, D. R. (1968) 'Rules, praise and ignoring: elements of elementary classroom control' Journal of Applied Behaviour Analysis, 1, 138-150

Mark, V. H. and Ervin, F. R. (1970) 'Violence and the brain' Harper and Row, Maryland

Megargee, E. I. (1966) 'Undercontrolled and over-controlled personality types in extreme anti-social aggression' Psychological Monographs, 80, Whole No. 611

Mikulas, W. L. (1972) 'Behaviour modification: an overview' Harper and Row, New York

Miller, N. (1941) 'The frustration-aggression hypothesis' Psychological Review, 48, 337-342

Mischel, W. (1968) 'Personality and Assessment' Wiley, New York

Moyer, K. E. (1971) 'The physiology of hostility' Markham, Chicago

Moyer, K. E. (1974) 'See differences in aggression' in R. C. Friedman, R. M. Riehart and R. C. Van de Wiele (eds.) 'Sex differences in behaviour', Wiley, New York

Moyer, K. E. (1976) 'The psychobiology of aggression Harper and Row, N. Y.

Nance, J. (1975) 'The Gentle Tasaday' Gollancz, London

Newberger, E. H. and Daniel, J. H. (1976) 'Knowledge and epidemiology of child abuse: a critical review of concepts' in R. Bourne and E. H. Newberger (eds.) Critical perspectives on child abuse, Lexington Books, Toronto

Novaco, R. W. (1978) 'Anger and coping with stress: cognitive behavioural interventions' in J. P. Foreyt and D. P. Rathsen (eds.) Cognitive Behaviour Therapy, Plenum, New York

N.S.P.C.C. (1976) 'At risk: report of the NSPCC Battered Child Research Team' Routledge, London

Olivier, B. (1977) 'The ventromedial hypothalamus and aggressive behaviour in rats' Aggressive Behaviour, 3, 47-56

Orr, J. (1984) 'Violence against women' Nursing Times, April 25, 34-36

Ounsted, C., Oppenheimer, R. and Lindsay, J. (1976) 'Aspects of bonding failure: the psychopathology and psychotherapeutic treatment of families of battered children' Developmental Medicine and Child Neurology, 16, 447-456

Owens, R. G. (1976) 'What do we think we are doing?' European Journal of Behavioural Analysis and Modification, 4, 214-220

Owens, R. G. (1979) 'Do psychologists need statistics?' Bulletin of the British Psychological Society, 32, 103-106

Owens, R. G. (1984) 'Psychological assessment' in P. McGuffin, M. Shanks and R. Hodgson (eds.) 'Scientific principles of psychopathology', Academic Press, London

Owens, R. G. and Ashcroft, J. B. (1982) 'Functional analysis in applied psychology' British Journal of Clinical Psychology, 21, 181-189

Owens, R. G. and Bagshaw, M. (1984) 'First steps in the functional analysis of aggression' in E. Karas (ed.) Current Issues in Clinical Psychology, Plenum, London

Packham, H. (1978) 'Managing the violent patient' Nursing Mirror, June 22, 17, 20.

Pahl, J. (1978) 'A Refuge for Battered Women' H.M.S.O., London

Paisnel, J. (1972) 'The Beast of Jersey' Robert Hale and Co., London

Patrick, J. (1973) 'A Glasgow gang observed' Eyre Methuen, London

Patterson, G. R., Cobb, J. A. and Ray, R. S. (1973) 'A social engineering technology for retraining the families of aggressive boys' in H. E. Adams and I. P. Unikel (eds.) Issues and trends in behaviour therapy, C. C. Thomas, Springfield, Illinois

Patterson, G. R., Littman, R. A. and Bricker, W. (1967) 'Assertive behaviour in children: a step towards a theory of aggression' Social Research Child Development Monograph, 32, 1-43

Phillips, E. L. (1968) 'Achievement place: token reinforcement procedures in a home-style rehabilitation setting for "pre-delinquent" boys' Journal of Applied Behaviour Analysis,

1, 213-223

Pinkston, E. M., Reese, N. H., LeBlanc, J. M. and Baer, D. M. (1973) 'Independent control of a preschool child's aggression and peer interaction by contingent teacher attention' Journal of Applied Behaviour Analysis, 6, 115-124

Pizzey, E. (1978) 'Scream quietly or the neighbours will hear' Pelican, Harmondsworth

Pizzey, E. and Shapiro, J. (1982) 'Prone to violence' Hamlyn, Middlesex

Powell, J., Martindale, A. and Kulp, S. (1976) 'An evaluation of time-sample measures of behaviour' Journal of Applied Behaviour Analysis, 8, 463-469

Price, W. H. (1978) 'Sex chromosome abnormalities in Special Hospital patients' in J. Gunn (ed.) "Sex offenders - a symposium", DHSS, London

Ransford, E. H. (1968) 'Isolation, powerlessness and violence: a study of attitudes and participation in the Watts riot' American Journal of Sociology, 73, 581-591

Reynolds, G. S., Catania, A. C. and Skinner, B. F. (1963) 'Conditioned and unconditioned aggression in pigeons' Journal of the Experimental Analysis of Behaviour, 6, 73-74

Rimm, D. C., de Groot, J. C., Boord, P., Heiman, J. and Dillow, P. V. (1971) 'Systematic desensitisation of an anger response' Behaviour Research and Therapy, 9, 273-380

Rogers, C. R. (On becoming a person; a therapist's view of psychotherapy' Constable, London

Rose, R. M., Gordon, T. P. and Bernstein, I. S. (1972) 'Plasma testosterone levels in the male rhesus: influence of sexual and social stimuli' Science, 178, 643-645

Rose, R. M., Holaday, J. W. and Bernstein, I. S. (1971) 'Plasma testosterone, dominance rank and aggressive behaviour in male rhesus monkeys' Nature, 231, 366-368

Sawa, M. Ueki, Y., Arita, M. and Harada, T. (1954) 'Preliminary report on the amydgaloidectomy on the psychotic patients with interpretation of oral emotional manifestations in schizophrenics' Folia Psychiatrica et Neurologia Japonica 7, 309-329.

Select Committee on Violence in Marriage (1975) First Report, H.M.S.O., London

Seligman, M. E. P. (1975) 'Helplessness: On Depression, Development and Death' W. H. Freeman and Co., San Francisco

Sheard, M. H. (1981) 'Shock-induced fighting (SIF):

psychopharmacological studies' Aggressive Behaviour, 7, 41-49

Shields, J. (1973) 'Heredity and psychological abnormality' in H. J. Eysenck (ed.) Handbook of Abnormal Psychology, Pitman Medical, London

Sidman, M. (1960) 'Tactics of Scientific Research' Basic Books, New York

Sipes, R. G. (1973) 'War, sports and aggression: an empirical test of two rival theories' American Anthropologist, 75, 64-85

Skinner, B. F. (1938) 'The Behaviour of Organisms' Appleton Century Crofts, New York

Skinner, B. F. (1953) 'Science and Human Behaviour' Macmillan, New York

Skinner, B. F. (1969) 'Contingencies of reinforcement' Appleton Century Crofts, New York

Skinner, B. F. (1971) 'Beyond freedom and Dignity' Knopf, New York

Slade, P. D. (1982) 'Towards a functional analysis of anorexia nervosa and bulimia nervosa' British Journal of Clinical Psychology, 21, 167-179

Smith, S. M. (1975) 'The Battered Child Syndrome' Butterworth, London

Stafford-Clark, D. (1967) 'What Freud Really Said' Penguin, Harmondsworth

Steele, B. F. and Pollock, C. B. (1968) 'A psychiatric study of parents who abuse infants and small children' in R. E. Helfer and C. H. Kempe (eds.) The Battered Child, University of Chicago Press, Chicago

Staumpfl, F. (1936) 'Die Urspringe des Verbrechens dargestellt am Lebenslauf von Zwillingen' Thieme, Leipzig

Sutherland, E.H. and Cressey, D. R. (1970) 'Criminology' 8th Edition, Lippincott, Philadelphia/New York/Toronto

Terrace, H. S. (1966) 'Stimulus control' in W. K. Honing (ed.) Operant Behaviour: areas of research and application' Appleton Century Crofts, New York

Terzian, H. and Ore, G. O. (1955) 'Syndrome of Kluver and Bucy reproduced in man by bilateral removal of the temporal lobes' Neurology 5, 373-380

Tharp, R. G. and Wetzel, R. J. (1969) 'Behaviour modification in the natural environment' Academic Press, New York

Thoresen, C. E. and Mahoney, M. J. (1968) 'Behavioural self-control' Holt, Rinehart and Winston, N. Y.

References

Ursin, H. (1981) 'Neuroanatomical Basis of
    Aggression' in P. F. Brain and D. Benton
    (eds.) 'Multidisciplinary Approaches to
    Aggression', Elsevier/North-Holland, Amsterdam
Ulrich, R. E. and Azrin, N. H. (1962) 'Reflexive
    fighting in response to aversive stimulation'
    Journal of the Experimental Analysis of
    Behaviour, 5, 511-520
Vadya, A. 'Expression and warfare among Swidden
    agriculturalists' American Anthropologist,
    63, 346-358
Vernon, W. and Ulrich, R. (1966) 'Classical
    conditioning of pain-elicited aggression'
    Science, 152, 668-669
Walker, N. (1968) 'Crime and Punishment in Britain'
    University Press, Edinburgh
Wallace, C. J., Teigen, J. R., Liberman, R. P. and
    Baker, V. (1973) 'Destructive behaviour
    treated by contingency contracts and
    assertive training: a case study' Journal of
    Behaviour Therapy and Experimental Psychiatry,
    4, 273-374
Walters, R. H. and Brown, M. (1963) 'Studies of
    reinforcement of aggression III: transfer of
    responses to an interpersonal situation'
    Child Development, 34, 563-571
Ward, M. H. and Baker, B. L. (1968) 'Reinforcement
    therapy in the classroom' Journal of Applied
    Behaviour Analysis, 1, 323-328
Yablonsky, L. (1962) 'The violent gang' Macmillan
Yalom, I., Green, R. and Fisk, N. (1973) 'Prenatal
    exposure to female hormones: effect on psycho-
    sexual development in boys' Archives of General
    Psychiatry, 28, 554-561
Zillman, D. (1979) 'Hostility and Aggression'
    Lawrence Erlbaum, New Jersey
Zillman, D., Bryant, J. and Sapolsky, B. S. (1978)
    'The enjoyment of watching sport contests' in
    J. Goldstine (ed.) Sports, Games and Play,
    Lawrence Erlbaum, New Jersey

195